THE
ALTERNATIVE
MEDICINE
SOURCEBOOK

THE ALTERNATIVE MEDICINE SOURCEBOOK

A Realistic Evaluation of Alternative Healing Methods

BY

STEVEN BRATMAN, M.D.

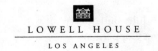

LOWELL HOUSE

LOS ANGELES

CONTEMPORARY BOOKS

CHICAGO

The purpose of this book is to educate. It is sold with the understanding that the author and Lowell House shall have neither liability nor responsibility for any injury caused or alleged to be caused directly or indirectly by the information contained in this book. While every effort has been made to ensure its accuracy, the book's contents should not be construed as medical advice. Each person's health needs are unique. To obtain recommendations appropriate to your particular situation, please consult a qualified health care provider.

Library of Congress Cataloging-in-Publication Data

Bratman, Steven.
    The alternative medicine sourcebook : a realistic evaluation of alternative healing methods / by Steven Bratman.
        p.   cm.
    Includes bibliographical references and index.
    ISBN 1-56565-626-1
    1. Alternative medicine—Popular works.   2. Self-care, Health.
    I. Title.
    R733.B75   1997
    615.5—dc21

                                                            96-49550
                                                            CIP

Requests for such permissions should be addressed to:
Lowell House
2020 Avenue of the Stars, Suite 300
Los Angeles, CA 90067

Lowell House books can be purchased at special discounts when ordered in bulk for premiums and special sales. Contact Department TC at the address above.

Publisher: Jack Artenstein
Associate Publisher, Lowell House Adult: Bud Sperry
Director of Publishing Services: Rena Copperman
Managing Editor: Maria Magallanes
Text design: Laurie Young
Illustrations: Sandy Nern

Manufactured in the United States of America
10 9 8 7 6 5 4 3 2 1

CONTENTS

This book is dedicated to my family,
Annie, Claire, and Jeshua,
and to my parents, Harvey and Marilyn.

INTRODUCTION

O nly a decade ago, alternative medicine in America was still a distinctly
countercultural phenomenon. But like the environmental movement (to
which it bears many similarities) alternative treatment has now become an established presence in mainstream culture. This progression may be due to many factors, from the maturation of the 1960s generation to the general decline in
respect for the medical establishment. Whatever the reason, alternative medicine
has come to wield a remarkable influence on health care delivery. The famous
1993 Eisenberg study reported in the *New England Journal of Medicine* estimated
that fully one-third of all Americans now use alternative treatments, spending billions of dollars every year in the process.

Information available about the field has grown along with public interest in
it. Nearly all the current literature, however, suffers from a lack of balance. The
typical alternative medicine book is evangelical, presenting alternative treatments
in glowing terms while disparaging conventional treatments as more a source of
illness than of health. If such a book critiques unconventional medicine at all, it
does so only in the mildest of terms.

The Alternative Medicine Sourcebook takes a unique position. It wholeheartedly affirms that alternative medicine can make a tremendous contribution to the search for health and healing, but counterbalances that appreciation with a substantive critique.

Such an evenhanded approach is more accurate and useful than mere praise. The various realms of unconventional treatment offer numerous techniques and insights that complement and in some cases clearly surpass the offerings of conventional medicine. The quality of alternative medicine as it is actually practiced, however, is highly inconsistent. Knowledge and nonsense, pragmatism and fantasy, and compassion and greed all coexist and intermingle, perhaps in equal measures. Those who wish to find help through alternative treatment must learn to distinguish between the worthwhile and the worthless.

Conventional medicine too has its good and its bad points. Common sense would say as much, for every human endeavor is imperfectly realized. Realistically, all approaches to healing possess a mixture of strengths and weaknesses. The strengths and weaknesses simply differ depending on the field in question.

This book takes a hard-boiled look at alternative medicine as it is practiced in real life. When it examines theories and ideals, it does so primarily to shed light on practical realities. Adopting a balanced attitude, it distinguishes between the best and the worst of available options.

Those who are presently trying to find their way through the complexities of alternative medicine options will find many valuable hints in the pages that follow. And others who have previously rejected alternative medicine because of its many faults may find a way to appreciate its particular, sometimes profound virtues.

SECTION I

A Realistic Look at Alternative Medicine

Some people are drawn to alternative medicine by a sense of affinity, but others come to it through desperation. Jim Humphries fell into the second category (all patient names in this book are pseudonyms). This thirty-four-year-old lawyer wanted my help for a strange collection of joint, muscle, and gut pains that had debilitated him for two years. Neither his primary care doctor nor any of the specialists to whom he had been sent had been able to diagnose the problem.

"My wife keeps telling me I should try alternative medicine," he explained. "And I can't think of anything else to do, so that's why I'm here." He didn't look happy.

"You're not too excited about it," I said, recognizing the signs. Whenever a spouse sends a patient for treatment, I have learned to expect trouble.

Jim folded his arms. "Actually, I'm not. I'm pretty skeptical."

"Me too," I said. "Alternative medicine is full of sloppy thinking, nonsense, faddishness, and commercialism. You should be skeptical."

Surprised by my answer, Jim continued in a softer voice. "Already I've been told to see a chiropractor, take something called malic acid, have my liver flushed out, get Rolfed, eat nothing but turkey and white rice, and I don't know what else. Everybody I know tells me what they think I should do, and everyone's advice is different. The chiropractor wanted me to come in three times a week for the rest of my life. I'm a lawyer. I'm used to things that make some rational sense. Someone said I should drink hydrogen peroxide, for God's sake!"

I replied, "Sounds like the chiropractor you visited is what I call the 'rack-'em, stack-'em, crack-'em type. Better chiropractic physicians do exist. You just have to know how to find them."

My prospective patient shook his head in disgust. "My medical doctor slammed his fist down when I said I planned to try alternative medicine, and he told me it was all garbage. I'm inclined to believe him, too—except for one thing: I hurt, and he can't help me."

"Here is how I look at it, Mr. Humphries," I replied. "I've been around alternative medicine for about twenty years, and in my opinion alternative medicine, just like everything else, is a mixed bag. It's not as bad as what medical doctors say about it and nowhere near as good as its proponents would have you believe. Alternative medicine does have a lot to offer. The challenge is separating the worthless from the useful, and then finding a method that will work for you."

He looked at me intently. "Well, how do I find the method that will work for me?"

All those who seek alternative treatment face the same question. There are so many contradictory options! Some sound good, at least on paper, while others appear to be absurd; regardless, each one can offer impressive testimonials of its worth. Unfortunately, there is no living expert who can point directly to the one method most likely to succeed in a particular case. The best any alternative practitioner can do is propose a handful of likely options and then resort to trial and error.

It was clear to me that Jim Humphries suffered from fibromyalgia. This is a fairly common condition but one that is little understood by medical science. It involves painful muscle knots and wandering areas of discomfort. Besides mild exercises and antidepressants, conventional medicine has little to suggest.

For its part, alternative medicine offers a wealth of conflicting choices: all the possibilities Jim recited and many more. While many treatments might have helped him, only a few had any great likelihood of doing so.

My short list included four options. Following my suggestions in succession, Jim tried three distinct treatments for fibromyalgia. Acupuncture helped him somewhat, supplement therapy failed altogether, and Feldenkrais brought him near-total recovery. He never tried the fourth—Chinese herbal treatment—because he didn't need to.

In subsequent pages, the reader will discover the information and insights necessary to find a way through the maze of alternative possibilities. The most important first step is to understand the nature of alternative medicine itself.

CHAPTER 1

What Is Alternative Medicine?

M ost proponents of the field would like to define alternative medicine as the art of using safe, natural methods to get to the root of problems, help the body to heal itself, and prevent diseases before they arise. While this definition sounds beautiful, it is pure romance. Alternative medicine seldom achieves such an idealized standard. The following pages paint a more realistic picture of the field.

Conventional physicians would describe alternative medicine somewhat differently, perhaps as a collection of unproved remedies, preposterous theories, and unsound practices of no value beyond what can be produced by the placebo effect. This unfriendly analysis is equally inaccurate.

The only true definition of alternative medicine is this minimalist one: Alternative medicine includes every available approach to healing that does not fall within the realm of conventional medicine.

Because it is only defined by what it is not, alternative medicine is an unregulated assortment of techniques, philosophies, and cultures of healing. Many patients assume that acupuncturists, chiropractors, naturopaths, and Rolfers all speak the same language and agree on a body of alternative principles, but this is a major misunderstanding. The various branches of alternative medicine frequently contradict one another. What links alternative practitioners is not a common philosophy but the attitude "any enemy of my enemy is my friend." In this case, it is conventional medicine that is the opponent.

For example, the naturopathic tradition urges all people to drink at least eight glasses of water daily. This practice is supposed to help flush out the kidneys. Indeed, some people find that this simple intervention promotes an enhanced sense of well-being and provides other tangible health benefits. So famous is this principle that many people regard it as established, incontrovertible fact.

Another popular health theory, however, the Japanese dietary system known as macrobiotics, urges people to drink only minimal amounts of water. Macrobiotic theorists back up their position with impressive arguments and testimonials. According to macrobiotic philosophy, drinking quarts and gallons of water is almost as harmful to your health as smoking cigarettes.

Both macrobiotics and the naturopathic kidney-flushing tradition belong to the general collection of ideas known as alternative medicine. Nevertheless, their thoughts on this subject (and on many others) directly contradict one another. They share the label of alternative medicine, not because they represent a single, coherent alternative position, but because neither one is embraced by conventional doctors.

The field is diverse and self-contradictory in many other ways. Most branches of alternative medicine, however, share at least a few unifying characteristics. It is important to understand these commonalities, because they are the source of both alternative medicine's strengths and its weaknesses.

THE THREE IDEALS
OF ALTERNATIVE MEDICINE

Most alternative practitioners are inspired by three great ideals: to provide treatment that is (1) natural, (2) holistic, and (3) promotes wellness. Conventional medicine largely lacks these aspirations. Even in alternative medicine, however, these wonderful ideals are far from fully achieved. Nonetheless, their mere presence as intentions gives alternative health care a distinctive mission and atmosphere.

Ideal #1 Natural Medicine

The first and most famous principle inspiring alternative practitioners is the ideal of natural medicine. Although it is hard to define precisely what the word *natural* means, its spirit is easy to recognize. The desire for natural treatment wells up from the same deep sources as the feelings that inspire the ecology movement. One person joins the Sierra Club, another prefers all-cotton clothing, and a third utilizes herbs. Such choices manifest a yearning for closer connection with nature, and they may collectively be described as the back-to-nature movement.

To many people, the modern world seems to have lost its way, substituting artificial reality for natural experience and replacing human rhythms with the electronic throbbing of machines. The back-to-nature phenomenon is a backlash against these changes. It is an attempt to bring back what is simple, original, and pure.

This is a movement driven far more by passion than by cold reasoning, although some reasoning supports it. For example, if a clothes shopper purchases a blouse from a catalog specializing in natural-fabric products, she does so because she anticipates feeling more wholesome wearing such clothes. Perhaps polyester doesn't "breathe" as well as cotton, nor wick body moisture as satisfactorily, but these are mere buttresses to a decision already made on aesthetic grounds. Cotton satisfies an instinct that polyester offends.

The same process operates in many aspects of the alternative medicine movement. Advocates of natural medicine prefer herbs over drugs, not because they have read formal risk/benefit analyses, but because to them a cup of ginger tea feels far more wholesome than any pharmaceutical product.

Indeed, alternative practitioners implicitly believe that herbs are meant to heal. At root, this is a spiritual inclination, a form of trust in providence.

The purified chemical prescriptions that come so easily to the hands of medical doctors seem, in contrast, on a par with pesticides, artificial fertilizers, red dye number three, and all the other toxic pollutants that afflict the world. Those who prefer natural treatments eye pharmaceuticals with some loathing, and, if they must take them, feel a bit polluted by doing so.

Most medical doctors simply do not understand such scruples. Doctors tend to feel an instinctive contempt for the very concept of "natural" substances. The form of medicine they practice aims to correct nature's errors, guard against nature's dangers, and supplement nature's weaknesses. To trust nature is not an ideal of conventional medicine.

Doctors do not believe that nature (or God) created herbs for the purpose of healing. To them, if an herb possesses medical benefits, it does so accidentally.

In other words, those who advocate natural medicine possess an aesthetic sensibility completely different from that of medical doctors. These two points of view reflect different emotional attitudes toward the world.

It is important to understand the ideal of natural medicine, because its presence guides the decisions of alternative practitioners inspired by it. For example, given the choice between a highly effective chemical antibiotic and a mildly effective herbal one, most alternative practitioners would choose the latter.

I recommend bearing this in mind when you evaluate claims made by proponents of alternative medicine. Authors and practitioners imbued with the dream of natural medicine may fail to pay much attention to results. In consequence, some of the treatments they propose do not work very well.

Some who turn to alternative medicine out of a search for natural treatment are eventually disappointed by the relative lack of concrete results. Of course, many natural treatments are quite effective, but not nearly as many as the idealistic books on herbs and whole foods would make it sound.

While the ideal of natural medicine inspires all alternative practitioners, it would be a mistake to believe that all branches of alternative medicine are "natural." Some are more natural than others. Herbal therapy and food medicine certainly deserve the title, as do therapeutic massage, the Feldenkrais method, Therapeutic Touch, and many others. However, numerous popular alternative methods aren't natural at all—but their proponents may hesitate to admit it.

Chelation therapy is a good example. This alternative treatment involves intravenous infusion of the chemical ethylenediaminetetraacetic acid. EDTA, as it is known for short, is a thoroughly artificial substance. It is not a regular part of the diet, nor does it grow in fields. Therefore, by any reasonable definition, EDTA chelation is not a natural therapy. Many other commonly accepted alternative treatments also require considerable stretches of the imagination to be considered natural.

Those who are interested in obtaining "natural" treatments may wish to avoid "unnatural" alternative options. When examining the major branches of alternative medicine in subsequent pages, I will point out those that fail to satisfy the natural medicine ideal.

Ideal #2 Holistic Medicine

Holism is another rallying cry of the alternative health movement. The extreme specialization of conventional medicine has caused many patients to seek out alternative practitioners who will see them as whole human beings.

Even among medical doctors, the remarkable nonholism of conventional medicine is a cause for rueful humor. I remember the case of a man who regularly visited six doctors: a urologist (for bladder problems), a cardiologist (for heart valve leakage), an ophthalmologist (for eye pain), a dermatologist (for skin lesions), an orthopedist (for bone degeneration), and a neurologist (for a minor stroke). What no one guessed—because they had never encountered the diagnosis in real life—was that this president of a major corporation suffered from late-stage syphilis. Every one of his symptoms stemmed from a single cause, but none of his specialists could put the whole picture together.

A retired doctor in the neighborhood finally made the diagnosis. He had seen many such cases in his youth. Fortunately, it was not too late to treat the patient. A course of penicillin produced a dramatic recovery from all his multitudinous symptoms.

Although mistakes as extreme as this one seldom occur, conventional medicine is always prone to the errors of specialization. This is an inevitable consequence of its scientific nature. Science is inherently analytical, breaking down wholes into slivers much better than it assembles slivers into wholes (although it does both).

As a part of science, conventional medicine excels at concentrating on isolated aspects of health, but it seldom reaches toward embracing the entire person. Individual doctors may try, but the methodology at which they are expert gives them no assistance in doing so. Rather than to step back and see the whole picture, medical training teaches doctors to zoom in on fine details. This fault is so connected to the fundamentals of the scientific method that it is not easy to suggest a remedy. Conventional medicine is probably doomed to ever-increasing specialization.

Unfortunately, this intrinsic lack of holism does not only lead to errors in treatment; it also wounds on an emotional and a spiritual level. Every modern individual already suffers from a lack of holism in daily life.

Modern life is terribly fragmented: into job and home, city and country, work and play, friends and strangers, body and mind, chores and pleasure, and quality time and wasted time. Many emotional illnesses stem from this texture of living, including depression, anxiety, and insomnia. Also, a number of important physical diseases are made worse by contemporary stresses. Heart disease, cancer, and infections all strike harder and more frequently at those whose social support structure is weak and whose level of stress is high.

If people are vaguely troubled when well, their vulnerabilities are intensified when they are sick. It is at the moment of illness that people most want to be understood as a whole. When they go to the doctor's office or the hospital and encounter the highly compartmentalized modern medical system, it may feel like insult added to injury.

In recognition of the overspecialization of conventional medicine, alternative medicine strives to deliver a more holistic form of healing. Many alternative practitioners make a sincere attempt to look at diet, emotions, and lifestyle as well as disease history; they try to treat stress as well as to prescribe herbs or supplements. This is especially true of those who practice acupuncture and Chinese medicine. The Chinese system weaves widely varying threads of human life experience into a single, whole-person diagnosis.

Alternative medicine is almost always more holistic than its conventional counterpart, and a visit to almost any alternative practitioner is more likely to be comforting and healing (on an emotional level) than a trip to the physician.

Nonetheless, alternative practitioners find that where holism is concerned, it is easier to set the table than to serve the meal. Human health and illness are subjects so vast that no one method or group of methods can encompass the whole. Even Chinese medicine, with its panoramic scope, can only address hundreds of details out of the billions of possibilities.

In fact, true holism is so difficult that some alternative practitioners don't even bother to attempt it. They may use methods that fragment the person nearly as much and in precisely the same ways as does conventional medicine. For example, a nutritionist may prescribe one supplement for frequent bladder infections, another for low blood sugar, and yet another for yeast infections. Is this holistic treatment? Not at all. Even acupuncturists, who are supposed to always think holistically, may fall back on symptomatic treatments out of laziness.

Still, alternative approaches to medicine tend to encourage practitioners to think holistically. Among the many alternative options, Chinese medicine, Ayurveda, and homeopathy are most wholeheartedly holistic.

Ideal #3 Wellness Promotion

When it comes to wellness promotion, alternative medicine has the field pretty much to itself. Alternative practitioners have made an essential insight: It is impossible to produce good health with drugs. Drugs prescribed by conventional physicians can fight illnesses, but they cannot produce a state of robust vitality.

In fact, most medical interventions produce a feeling of vague discomfort rather than of health. The majority of drugs cause at least one of the following side effects: malaise, drowsiness, headache, stomach upset, insomnia, dry mouth, or sexual dysfunction. Ordinarily, a medical treatment solves one problem at the cost of creating other, hopefully lesser ones; seldom does a drug make a patient "feel like a million bucks."

The immediate effects of alternative treatment are generally quite the opposite. Acupuncture produces a sense of pleasant relaxation, chiropractic a feeling of more energy, and vitamin supplementation the expectation of better health. Of course, part of these effects may be attributed to positive suggestion, but even that is an important difference: People so strongly expect drugs to make them feel ill that placebo pills do so as well. In other words, all drugs communicate a negative placebo effect on top of their actual side effects. Conversely, natural treatments suggest health and well-being.

Furthermore, conventional medicine does not focus its energy on thinking up ways to enhance overall good health. The concept of good health is simply too nebulous for medical science to engage. Instead, conventional medical practice orbits around diseases, using unpleasant and often humiliating tests and treatments to ward them off or to conquer them. In contrast, the primary thrust of many alternative methods is to strengthen the individual.

Both these approaches are valuable, but in different circumstances. To clarify this distinction, I like to use the image of "strong tigers versus weak legs." When a tiger bites a person's leg, the cause of the problem is a strong tiger—not a weak leg! Removing the tiger is the best solution.

On the other hand, if a person's legs are unsteady, he may constantly bark his shins on coffee tables. External factors are not the actual cause of his injuries—the real problem lies in the weakness of his legs. Removing every piece of furniture, while it might cut down on bruises, would miss the point.

Some illnesses resemble the first pattern most closely, others the second. For example, AIDS is a classic "tiger" illness. No matter how good a person's health, if he is exposed to the HIV virus often enough he will almost certainly succumb to the disease. The best way to prevent this infection is to avoid exposure.

Bacterial pneumonia and bubonic plague are also "tiger" illnesses. The infectious organisms involved are so powerful that many individuals' immune systems cannot defeat them. Antibiotics help make victory possible by killing or weakening the bacteria involved. They do nothing to strengthen the immune system itself.

In contrast, sinus infections are "weak leg" illnesses. Whether or not a person develops infectious sinusitis depends more on personal factors than on the presence or absence of germs. The viruses and bacteria that cause sinus infections are very prevalent. A person develops a sinus infection, not so much because she is exposed to germs, but because of conditions within herself. In this case, hunting after "tiger" germs with the gun of antibiotics is less than ideal. It does nothing to prevent future infections. The optimum treatment would be to promote robust immunity. However, there are few techniques available in conventional medicine to accomplish this goal.

Most of the time, conventional medicine focuses its attention on tigers, which it calls pathogens. It pays relatively little attention to strengthening legs—in other words, to improving the immune system. As explained previously, this is a natural consequence of the Western scientific method. Science always seeks to break down complex systems into simpler elements. External causes are easier to identify than subtle problems in the body as a whole.

In contrast, various forms of alternative medicine are primarily oriented toward the "weak legs" side of the equation. These systems devote considerable attention to improving the body's state of balance and increasing its natural strength. They do not succeed at this intention nearly as well as they would like, but at least they make the attempt.

"Tonic herbs" are one kind of wellness-promoting technique used in alternative medicine. Herbs such as ginseng (China), suma (Brazil), and gentian (Europe) are used to strengthen one or another body system. Dr. Andrew Weil, one of the leading exponents of alternative medicine, has pointed out that there are no equivalents to tonic herbs in Western medicine. Asthma medications reduce bronchial inflammation, but they do not promote strong lungs. As soon as the medication is stopped, the symptom returns. In contrast, tonic herbs function more like exercise and good nutrition: they are intended to improve health in a way that will last even after the herb is stopped.

The two great Eastern medical systems of Chinese medicine and Ayurveda use a more sophisticated approach. While these systems do employ tonic herbs, they use them only as part of an integrated approach that involves many methods.

Other alternative medical techniques also aim at promoting good health, such as those used by chiropractors, naturopaths, and homeopaths. The same can be said for meditation, tai chi, yoga, prayer, healthy venting of emotions, ocean air, mountain air, laughter, following your bliss, drinking Kombucha tea, eating super blue-green algae, and avoiding doctors altogether. A cartload of nonsense is mixed in with the considerable truth behind these widely varying claims.

In real life, overall lifestyle changes produce an improvement in the sense of well-being more frequently than any specialized alternative modalities. There are exceptions, however. Every week I meet patients who swear that one or another technique has made them altogether more healthy. Sometimes these responses are short-lived and may be attributed more to enthusiasm for a new idea than to any actual change. But quite a few prove to be solid and long-lasting.

There is no way to predict in advance which method will work best for a given individual. Trial and error are inescapable here, as in most aspects of alternative treatment.

Whatever method you use, I suggest avoiding the "new convert" syndrome. Don't try to talk all your friends and relatives into doing what you are doing until you've stuck with the process for at least a year. Many new health ideas fizzle. But if you are still enthusiastic long after the novelty has worn off, then your seasoned advice may truly benefit a neighbor.

HOW WELL ARE
THESE IDEALS PRACTICED?

Although these three great ideals inspire all those involved with alternative medicine, not every branch of alternative medicine makes an equally serious attempt to actualize them. Figure 1-1 evaluates a variety of methods from this perspective.

Generally, the more ideals a modality manifests, the more respect it deserves as a truly alternative treatment. The subsequent sections devoted to the various branches of alternative medicine will explore the extent to which these ideals are actually achieved in each field.

Besides the three ideals, three other characteristics pervade alternative medicine: a belief in vitalism, a tendency toward romanticism, and a stance that may be described as the underdogs versus the authorities.

Figure 1-1

Branches of alternative medicine and their actualization of three ideals: naturalness, holism, and wellness promotion.

	Natural	**Holistic**	**Wellness**
Acupuncture	?	yes	yes
Chinese Herbs	yes	yes	yes
Chiropractic	yes	?	yes
Feldenkrais	yes	no	yes
Massage	yes	?	yes
Body/Mind	yes	no	yes
Western Herbs	yes	no	yes
Dietary Therapy	yes	yes	yes
Supplement Medicine	no	no	yes
Chelation Therapy	no	no	no
Super H_2O_2, etc.	no	no	yes

Note: The category named "Wellness" refers to an intention to promote wellness, not necessarily success at achieving it.

Vitalism

Nearly all varieties of alternative medicine believe in the existence of a "life energy" or "vital force." Conventional medicine certainly does not agree. Science supposes itself to have disproved the concept of vitalism centuries ago. To medical doctors, the body is no more and no less than a complex machine.

But to most alternative practitioners, the existence of a vital force is obvious and fundamental. For them, healing consists not in fighting diseases but in assisting the vital force to do its work. Wellness is essentially a state where the energy of life flourishes. Disease is a condition where vitality is blocked.

Traditional herbalists are vitalistic when they say that herbs contain a healing virtue. So are those who advocate raw foods in the diet, in the belief that uncooked fruits and vegetables "are more alive." In Chinese medicine, the applicable term is Qi (pronounced "chee"), an energy that is seen as flowing through every cell of the body. Acupuncture is supposed to correct stagnation, deficiencies, and local excesses of Qi. More than simply learning facts, acupuncturists try to sensitize themselves to interact with that energy.

Almost every branch of alternative medicine espouses a belief in vital energy. But, in real life, this philosophy has no effect on the practices of some alternative practitioners. A surprising amount of what is called alternative medicine consists of treatments applied just as mechanically as any conventional intervention. Furthermore, while medical doctors would never use the phrase "life force," some conventional methods do focus on assisting the body's own healing process. These exceptions to the general rule will be described in more detail later.

Romanticism

Alternative practitioners are usually more romantically idealistic than conventional medical doctors. Inspired and uplifted by the three high ideals and the vitalistic attitude just described, many approach their work with a sense of reverence and awe. They feel that by practicing alternative medicine they are bringing positive spiritual values into the world.

This romanticism, however, has a dark side. Alternative practitioners too often develop such extreme love for their beliefs that they become ideologues, caring far more for principles than for actualities. This can lead to a kind of religious faith in the efficacy of a treatment and the development of extreme views.

An example may be found in acupuncture. While most acupuncturists are pragmatists and look for tangible results from treatment, some seem to believe that acupuncture in itself is a blessing to the patient. Even if their services fail, excessively idealistic acupuncturists may smugly believe that they have performed a genuine service. I have often heard such practitioners say: "I'm sure that acupuncture helped my patient at some level. Maybe it will stop him from getting cancer." This is a fault peculiar to alternative healing professionals; medical doctors do not usually believe that their mere presence is a grace.

I recommend evaluating a prospective practitioner to make sure he or she actually pays attention to results. Reality-based practitioners admit both successes and failures, and acknowledge that theories with which they work are not all-powerful and all-wise.

Another common consequence of alternative medicine's idealism is the development of extreme viewpoints. For example, vegetarianism develops into nondairy (lacto-ovo) vegetarianism, which in turn grows into "fruitarianism," (eating only fruit) and, in its final evolution, "breatharianism"—the belief that it is possible and desirable to live on air alone (I am not kidding!). In every aspect of alternative medicine there is a marked tendency to carry principles toward infinity.

I caution people to avoid being seduced by extreme philosophies. In my opinion, health consists above all in an enhanced state of balance, not in radical departures from it.

Underdogs versus the Authorities

Another general characteristic of alternative medicine deserves discussion: its disposition to adopt an attitude of knee-jerk rebelliousness. In other words, alternative practitioners tend to believe that everything conventional medicine proposes is wrong, while everything opposed by the American Medical Association (AMA) must be true.

Democrats behave similarly when Republicans control Congress, and vice versa. Those who lack power always snipe at those in authority. In Western society, medical doctors dominate health care, while alternative practitioners endure a perpetual state of powerlessness and marginalization. The latter's natural state, therefore, is rebellion.

A good example may be found in the history of fluoridation. Enthusiastic antifluoride campaigns have been part of the alternative medicine scene ever since fluoridation began. The only reason behind this protest is the fact that conventional medicine invented the treatment. If it hadn't, every health food store would undoubtedly sell fluoride products! One can buy selenium, chromium, vanadium, manganese, boron, and many other peculiar mineral supplement in such stores. Why not fluoride?

This policy of opposition for opposition's sake makes for strange bedfellows. For example, there is a full-fledged alternative cult around the antiepilepsy drug Dilantin. As a treatment for seizures, alternative medicine proponents condemn Dilantin, but at the same time they extol its virtues as an uncomventional cure for dozens of other diseases. This makes no rational sense; it is just part of the typical geography of rebellion.

Feelings of powerlessness frequently cause alternative health advocates to indulge in conspiracy theories. Thus many of my friends and colleagues believe that medical doctors deliberately prescribe tests and treatments that create sickness in order to assure themselves future business. I strenuously disagree: doctors may be arrogant but they are not malicious. Similar fantasies regard pharmaceutical companies, who are supposed to be in league with the Food and Drug Administration (FDA), the AMA, and, no doubt, the seven evil men who secretly rule the world. Drug companies, it is said, build in side effects in order to sell drugs to treat those side effects.

In my opinion, partisan claims like these are an impediment to clear thinking and an obstacle to optimum care. I take a different view: that conventional medicine is a mixture of good and bad. Its practitioners are motivated partly by compassion and partly by base motives, and its practices are founded both on fact and on politics. Much the same may be said of the various branches of alternative medicine.

Every healer is fallible and influenced by personal prejudices. I recommend that patients gather as much information as possible, trust no one entirely, and reserve the right to make all final decisions.

THE TWO TYPES OF ALTERNATIVE MEDICINE

So far I have been discussing those qualities that apply to all branches of alternative medicine. At this point, however, there is a major juncture of roads. The world of alternative treatments divides neatly into two distinct categories: those that attempt to function as forms of science, and others that may be best described as nonscientific crafts.

The Semiscientific Approaches

In this category may be found some of the most popular alternative methods, such as the therapeutic uses of herbal extracts, vitamins, and food supplements. All these methods are backed to some degree by scientific analysis and clinical trials. In recent years, the quality and breadth of this research has improved dramatically, however, much of it still remains unsatisfactory.

Medical researchers require a fairly high level of science before they will endorse a new drug. Alternative practitioners, on the other hand, are willing to embrace herbs and supplements when the evidence backing their use is still fairly incomplete. For this reason, the science behind these semi-scientific branches of alternative medicine is spotty and often a bit speculative.

Conventional medicine itself has many unscientific aspects. But there is a major difference of degree. The more scientific branches of alternative medicine still have a long way to go to reach the admittedly imperfect science practiced by medical doctors.

It is important to bear this in mind when considering statements made by alternative practitioners. Although they may use scientific words, their reliability in hard fact is generally lower than the language may seem to imply. Indeed, the partially scientific branches of alternative medicine are haunted by what I call "pretend science." I am referring to methods that use impressive-sounding words and phrases with no real science underlying them.

This practice, nearly ubiquitous in the semiscientific forms of alternative medicine, is fundamentally dishonest. It lowers the reputation of alternative medicine and is responsible for much of the hostility conventional physicians feel toward alternative practitioners. Worse, fancy language can mislead people into believing that they are buying a scientifically reputable product. Health food store shelves are full of product literature that sounds splendid but doesn't really mean anything.

So fertile is the mind, and so complex are the processes of the body, that anyone with the capacity for associative thinking can invent a scientific-sounding theory. For this reason, it is important not to be easily impressed by product literature. Some of it is reliable, but much of it is simply commercial tripe.

In later pages, I attempt to help the reader identify the more reliable forms of semiscientific alternative medicine.

The Healing Arts

The other major category of alternative approaches to healing principally includes acupuncture and Chinese medicine, the various bodywork arts (such as massage), and the alternative psychotherapies. Lacking any scientific foundation and admitting it willingly, such approaches to healing possess the virtues and limitations of crafts. These are the most profoundly alternative aspects of alternative medicine, and (when practiced well) its most significant and highest forms.

The semiscientific methods just mentioned retain much of the "look and feel" of science. Like conventional medicine, they involve pills—just different pills. The most solidly validated and potent of these pills often migrate into the mainstream medical world. But healing crafts employ methods, philosophies, and skills entirely different from those of conventional medicine.

The healing arts offer a human touch in a world where medicine is dominated by chemicals and machines. Science is mechanistic, rigid, and preoccupied with weighing and measuring. In contrast, many healing arts use subtle and refined skills of the hand and eye that are difficult, if not impossible, to quantify.

The Feldenkrais method is one such healing art. In my experience, this wonderful movement therapy is far more effective for treating musculoskeletal pain than anything conventional medicine has to offer. However, there is no chance it will be incorporated into conventional practice. It is simply too subjective, too much an art.

Feldenkrais practitioners work wordlessly, using fluid hands-on methods that cannot be standardized. Science is incapable of dealing with methods such as these; it needs to reduce to fundamentals everything it studies—to measure, weigh, and analyze down to atoms. But, freed from the need to be so left-brained, alternative practitioners may become like fine artists: they can become healers.

The word *healer* has many possible meanings. In the sense I use it here, a healer is one who works with sensitivity and craft to encourage a deep healing process. Medical doctors rarely function in this way. They simply apply standardized protocols and, waiting for the arrival of defined checkpoints, hope for the best. Modern medicine allows little leeway for craft, artistry, or intuition.

Doctors are primarily intelligent technicians, and if the field continues on its present path, they may soon be replaceable (to a large extent) by computers. One of my medical school instructors stated this as an explicit goal: "Our objective is to get the hunches out of medicine. We need to know exactly what we're doing, rather than rely on our feelings."

In contrast, healers use "feel" and intuition in their work. Subjective sensations and experiences are just as important to them as are objective facts. Like master cabinetmakers, advanced bodyworkers learn to think with their fingers, understanding nuances of touch that could never be put into words. This type of skill is vanishing from scientific medicine.

Sometimes crafts can accomplish what science cannot even attempt. Consider Stradivarius, who constructed his wonderful violins without troubling to discover the precise mechanism by which particular resins and woods amplify sound vibrations. He used no microscopes, tension gauges, or synthesized varnishes. What he did with his ears, hands, hard work, and inspiration cannot be duplicated by any scientist nor by all the technology available in the modern world. Similarly, the linear, scientific methods of medical doctors cannot always create healing techniques to match the best offerings of alternative medicine.

Compared to conventional medicine's measured mixtures of electrolytes, the better alternative healing arts are like fine wines. They possess a depth and subtlety science cannot match. When a practitioner of a mature field such as acupuncture, cranial osteopathy, or the Feldenkrais method reaches a certain level of development, she may begin to provide a service conventional medicine (and the semiscientific branches of alternative medicine) can scarcely comprehend.

In this regard, alternative practitioners share a predicament with other craftsmen: the twentieth century is not the golden age of crafts. In products, as well as in medicine, we have learned to make do with standardized offerings. This is a great loss. Fortunately, not all crafts are gone from the world, and in alternative medicine, as elsewhere, what remains can offer much.

In later chapters, I point out which branches of alternative medicine involve the highest levels of craft.

Artistic License

Craftspeople frequently use metaphors to help them in their work. In the 1970s I worked briefly as an unskilled assistant to a cabinetmaker. One day, when I was damaging a good piece of walnut in an attempt to sand it, he looked over my shoulder and shook his head. "See how angry that grain is?" he asked. "When grain is that angry, you must approach it tactfully." He then showed me the proper sanding technique, involving gentle, short strokes.

This master craftsperson did not really attribute emotions to wood. When he described the grain as "angry," he meant that its swirls and whorls were of a particular type. Conceptualizing that pattern as "angry" was useful poetry. The carpenter's metaphor helped me to do a better job.

Similarly, alternative practitioners feel free to speak loosely and think in wide strokes. This liberty from literal reality is both helpful and problematic. Their freedom allows alternative practitioners to explore the most profound avenues of healing art. However, they may also fall under the spell of fanciful speculations, unbalanced ideologies, and irresponsible conjectures.

The healing arts would perhaps benefit if its practitioners incorporated a little more science as a reality check. Double-blind controlled experiments would not be necessary. Systematic and impartial interviews of patients after a course of treatment would be sufficient. However, few alternative therapists have the interest or the skills necessary to conduct a proper scientific investigation. Their gifts are artistic and intuitive. That is why they became alternative practitioners in the first place, rather than medical doctors.

For this reason, it is important not to take literally everything spoken by practitioners of healing arts. Their words should be understood more in broad terms than in specifics. Scientific branches of medicine are far more precise, but less open to intuition and subtle craft. It's an inescapable trade-off. I also recommend paying close attention to whether a particular alternative craftsperson actually produces quality work. Those who are often unsuccessful, whether carpenters or chiropractors, should be fired. But those who function at a high level of competence should be enthusiastically recommended to others.

In all its forms, from semiscientific techniques to subtle healing arts, alternative medicine includes much that is useful and effective. Sometimes its methods are more effective than the standard approaches of conventional medicine, or they produce equally good results with fewer side effects. But these contributions can be difficult to discern amid the many myths surrounding unconventional treatment. The next chapter attempts to dispel some of the most common misconceptions, in order to make it easier to appreciate what is truly useful about alternative medicine.

CHAPTER 2

Alternative Medicine:
Myths and Realities

O ne of the first discoveries everyone makes when exploring alternative medicine is that this field is dominated by extreme and grandiose claims. Some of these come from within the field, and are full of praise. Others come from alternative medicine's critics, who have almost nothing nice to say about a field they regard as worse than useless. But, actually, everyone is shouting half-truths.

In this section, I analyze the statements most commonly made regarding alternative medicine. By carefully separating myths and reality, I hope to help you arrive at a clear understanding of the actual nature and uses of alternative medicine.

CLAIM: Alternative Medicine Helps the Body to Heal Itself
(while conventional medicine only attacks diseases).

ANALYSIS: To most proponents of alternative medicine, this is a self-evident statement. It is repeated in books and magazine articles, on talk shows and in the offices of a thousand practitioners. There is some truth to it. Alternative practitioners definitely focus more on strengthening the body as a whole than do conventional physicians.

For example, consider a bacterial infection of the skin, such as staphylococcal boils. An herbalist might recommend echinacea for the purpose of activating the person's immune system. In the same situation, a medical doctor might prescribe the antibiotic dicloxacillin. Such treatment wouldn't support the body—it would just kill the bacteria.

Similarly, for a patient with angina, a nutritionist would likely recommend a no-fat diet; a cardiologist might propose balloon dilation of the arteries feeding the heart. Alternative practitioners often recommend methods intended to permit the body to heal its own troubles in its own ways. In contrast, conventional doctors generally prefer to intervene forcefully and dramatically. This dichotomy characterizes the different tendencies of alternative and conventional practitioners.

These tendencies are not absolute, however. Many popular alternative methods attack diseases just as forcefully as does conventional medicine. For example, there is currently a huge interest in the common yeast known as *Candida*. Many books and thousands of alternative practitioners recommend dietary changes, supplements, and various drugs to inhibit this organism's growth. While this may be good medicine (a proposition that is open to dispute), it certainly isn't helping the body to heal itself. How does attacking yeast with caprylic acid differ conceptually from destroying bacteria with dicloxacillin? Both focus on killing a pathogen rather than on supplementing the body's inherent strength. Alternative practitioners seldom point out this discrepancy between advertisement and reality.

Further diluting the distinction, many aspects of conventional medicine rely to a great extent on the body's own healing powers. The antibiotic tetracycline is a good example: it does not kill bacteria directly, but simply inhibits the organisms' growth. The battle must be won by the individual's immune system.

The modern treatment of wounds shows the same point even better. After years of experimenting with various creams, ointments, and salves, orthodox medical doctors have come to believe that the best way to heal a wound is to do no more than keep it clean and exposed to the air. The body heals the wound itself; the doctor's job is simply to make sure no foreign particles interfere. Such treatment is natural medicine at its most elemental, and on a par with the highest of alternative ideals.

Thus, the distinction heading this section is not altogether accurate. Alternative medicine does not always help the body heal itself, nor does conventional medicine depend on its own interventions alone. Nonetheless, on average, alternative medicine slants more toward enhancing the body's strength, and conventional medicine toward treating diseases.

CLAIM: Alternative Medicine Prevents Illness
(while conventional medicine only treats diseases once they occur).

ANALYSIS: As described in the previous chapter, many alternative techniques aim at promoting wellness. A robustly healthy person is much less likely to get sick; therefore, wellness promotion is preventive medicine.

Alternative medical practitioners have made many significant contributions to prevention. It was naturopaths, not medical doctors, who originally pushed low-fat vegetarian diets. In those days, medical authorities ridiculed the idea. Now, we know that such a diet drastically reduces the risk of nearly all major diseases of later life. Similarly, it was nutritionists, not M.D.s, who first promoted antioxidants. Today, even major medical journals extol the (still theoretical) preventive virtues of vitamins E, A, and C.

To show how strongly alternative medicine focuses on prevention, proponents often tell the following story: Long ago, it is said, acupuncturists were paid only when a patient was well. Patients who became sick were entitled to free treatment, and patients and their entire families could even move into the acupuncturist's house for the duration of the illness. Sickness was considered a sign that the doctor had failed. Modern doctors, the story continues, only treat sick people, which shows how inferior they are to the ancients.

This is a very nice tale. However, an important detail is usually left out: The acupuncturist in the legend was granted a great deal of authority along with his retainer. He was given the right to dictate every morsel of food that passed through his patients' lips, require hours of daily exercises, insist on particular living conditions (whether hot or cold, dry or damp), and control many other aspects of his patients' lives. Those patients who failed in any of these instructions thereby let the acupuncturist off the hook. Not many Americans would willingly submit themselves to so much regulation!

And that's the rub: No amount of alternative treatment can promote wellness in patients who do not take care of themselves. Frequently, people come to me who can't find the time to exercise, are reluctant to quit smoking cigarettes, and love to eat hamburgers—but they want me to give them vitamins to keep them well! When I tell them it's impossible without major lifestyle changes, they get angry.

In fact, the most effective preventive techniques in existence are already at the disposal of every individual who chooses to use them: regular aerobic exercise, abstention from cigarettes and other poisons, a semivegetarian diet, and good stress management. Universal adoption of these simple prescriptions would undoubtedly do far more to improve the overall health of Americans than all the interventions of all the doctors in practice, alternative and conventional combined.

Doctors can't change people's lifestyles for them. They can provide education, but most people already know what to do; the lack is in the doing, not the knowing. Moreover, even people whose lifestyles are impeccable get sick. I know many people who live clean lives, get regular acupuncture treatments, take herbs, practice tai chi, and reside deep in the country to escape pollutants. Nonetheless, they still catch colds and develop other diseases to which humans are susceptible.

Perhaps regular acupuncture (or other alternative treatment) cuts down on the incidence of future problems, but that is a hypothesis very difficult to verify. Alternative practitioners are usually filled with idealism about their chosen methods. Many believe implicitly that their work safeguards their patients' futures. Unfortunately, practitioner confidence is not enough. Research results would help, but virtually none are available. Many of alternative medicine's supposed preventive powers are likely just optimistic fantasies.

Some aspects of alternative medicine undoubtedly do provide prevention. Undergoing yoga practice or Feldenkrais training appears to minimize the frequency of future injuries; cutting out milk appears to substantially reduce the incidence of colds; and taking large doses of vitamin E probably reduces the risk of heart attack. Prevention is real, it is simply difficult to achieve and to verify.

For this reason, conventional medicine has historically paid more attention to treating illnesses as they arise than to preventing them. Medical doctors try hard not to indulge in unfounded optimism. For a preventive technique to be accepted by scientific medicine, its effectiveness has to be documented by solid research. But it takes years and millions of dollars to prove that a treatment cuts down on future problems. It is much easier to document "overnight successes."

Nonetheless, it was medical doctors, not alternative practitioners, who discovered the link between high blood pressure, high cholesterol, and heart disease. Medical doctors invented vaccines, which are certainly intended as prevention (even if some alternative practitioners take exception to them). And it was scientific medicine that was largely responsible for the most successful disease prevention effort of all time: sanitation. When medical researchers discovered disease-producing germs, they catalyzed what was then called the National Sanitation movement. The results included effective sewage disposal and safer food and water. No doubt these interventions have prevented far more illnesses than any other intentional health care measure in history.

Again, it is clear that the distinction made in this proposition is not absolute. No form of medicine has a monopoly on prevention.

CLAIM: Alternative Medicine Treats Causes
(while conventional medicine is no more than a Band-Aid approach).

ANALYSIS: This is a war cry frequently shouted by proponents of alternative medicine. But it too is only a partial truth.

Conventional medicine definitely focuses more on symptoms than on causes. This is not due to any tenet of faith among doctors (who would much rather treat the root of problems); it is simply a by-product of real life. Almost always it is easier to alleviate symptoms than to remedy causes. This is true in every field, from social work to international policymaking, in the inner city and in sub-Saharan Africa.

Alternative practitioners also find it difficult to address causes, but they have many more options available to them than their conventional counterparts. Medical doctors are limited to scientifically verified methods, whereas alternative therapists can try almost whatever they please. Sometimes it is easier to find the root of a problem by art than by science.

A good example of this may be seen in the treatment of chronic muscular pain. Doctors are superb at repairing broken bones, they get passing marks at removing bulging intervertebral disks, but they are virtually helpless in the face of soft-tissue pain. When nothing shows on X ray, but the patient still hurts, what's a doctor to do?

The doctor can offer anti-inflammatory medications and other pain relievers. Unfortunately, such drugs don't treat chronic pain very successfully. As one patient said to me, "Prescribing ibuprofen for my bad back is like recommending vodka for a bad marriage. It may dull the symptoms, but it will not address any of the real problems." Physical therapy is not much better, consisting of little more than glorified hot packs and unproved exercise methods.

When a true bodywork art such as Rolfing or Feldenkrais is compared against these conventional approaches, medicine's methods truly seem to deserve the Band-Aid label. A sophisticated bodyworker delves deeply into the causes of pain, increases awareness, overcomes blocks, works to release bad habits, and helps to create good ones. Conventional medical methods primarily just dull pain. The various bodywork arts are so much more effective at treating musculoskeletal pain that in comparison conventional treatment is no real treatment at all.

There are many more such examples. On average, alternative medicine seeks a deeper level of treatment than does conventional medicine.

Not all alternative methods are equally deep, however. Many are as superficial as the typical conventional treatment. Taking glucosamine sulfate (a food supplement) for joint pain or cranberry juice for bladder infections are two alternative Band-Aids that come to mind. Neither one addresses the causes behind the symptom it treats.

Ultimately, no treatment corrects the cause of illness. Beneath each cause lies a deeper cause, and below that, a still deeper one, descending all the way to the unchangeable fact of mortality.

For example, consider a patient who suffers from frequent bacterial sinus infections. The most symptomatic treatment imaginable might involve using decongestants to treat the patient's stuffy nose. This would not eradicate the bacteria, speed healing, or prevent future infections, but it might provide some temporary relief.

To go a little deeper, a medical doctor might prescribe an antibiotic to kill the bacteria. An appropriately chosen drug would probably cure one particular sinus infection, but it wouldn't prevent future ones. This is as far as conventional medicine can go. It is not the doctor's fault that she or he does nothing more. Medical science simply does not know how to prevent sinus infections.

A naturopath would ask the deeper question: Why is this patient so susceptible to infection? She might theorize that food allergies have caused a buildup of mucus. Mucus provides a convenient nutrient base for germs to grow in. Therefore, if the patient identifies and avoids allergenic foods, she will produce less mucus and, hopefully, develop fewer sinus infections. This is a common stopping point for alternative practitioners who are interested in nutrition.

But what caused the patient to develop food allergies? This, the next deeper question, is seldom considered by naturopaths. To counsel mere avoidance of certain foods is simply to treat the surface of the condition. A truly deep treatment would seek to eliminate the cause of allergies. Otherwise, what is to stop new allergies from developing?

Too often, that is precisely what happens. While I have seen many people improve their health through avoiding triggering foods, the process seems to have no end. Over time it becomes necessary to eliminate more and more items from the diet. Each slight dietary indiscretion leads to a host of dire consequences. Patients become increasingly sensitive and obsessed, eventually reaching a point where every sniffle, every trifling ache, every marital conflict, and each poor grade at school can be attributed to a single raisin or pinto bean consumed in violation of the law. In the end, although the patient may be living on turkey, white rice, and hypoallergenic vitamins, all the symptoms recur, and she is then both sick and deprived.

Chinese medicine offers a means of going one level deeper. To cure the very state of being allergic, an acupuncturist might try to "strengthen the spleen energy." According to Chinese medical theory, a condition called "deficient spleen Qi" can cause numerous symptoms, including food allergies, fatigue, hypoglycemia, depression, unclear thinking, frequent infections, and poor digestion. Certain acupuncture points and appropriate herbs are supposed to correct this condition, thereby solving the problem at its root.

But is it truly the root? How did the "spleen Qi" become weak in the first place? If this is not understood, isn't it possible that the spleen, even if strengthened, might grow weak again?

There is no end to this process. The chain of causation goes on forever. The ultimate cause of illness is physical mortality itself and the flaws, contradictions, and imperfections of life on earth.

Nonetheless, there is a movement toward wholeness that can be recognized when it occurs. By great leaps or a slow crawl, individuals move from suffering into new states of balance. The best alternative practitioners seek to promote such profound growth. Because it takes a certain greatness of soul to understand the need, healers who endeavor to provide deep healing are rare and precious. Those who are successful are even rarer.

CLAIM: Alternative Medicine Is Cost-effective.

ANALYSIS: This statement simply isn't true, for one reason: craftwork is always more expensive than mass-produced products. Alternative medicine is labor-intensive. Properly performed acupuncture, chiropractic, Feldenkrais, or Rolfing, to name a few important methods, ordinarily require lengthy visits repeated over extended periods of time. Furthermore, these sessions usually require the undivided attention of the practitioner. Compared to such treatments, drugs are cheap!

Even the simple alternative forms, such as food supplement therapy, are fairly pricey. Many patients have brought me grocery bags full of the expensive supplements their naturopath or nutritionist has prescribed. Few are inexpensive individually, and collectively the total bill can add up to hundreds of dollars each month.

Of course, conventional medicine is extremely expensive too. Nongeneric drugs can cost upward of fifteen dollars a pill, and the complex services of a modern hospital may ring up thousands of dollars a day. Surgery especially is terribly expensive, both in direct costs and in time lost from work. Whenever an alternative treatment such as chiropractic can substitute for surgery, patients will undoubtedly save money, and probably experience a better outcome as well.

However, a direct cost comparison between alternative and conventional medicine is not entirely fair. Part of the cost difference is due to health insurance. Because someone else (the insurer) pays for prescription drugs and other conventional medical services, there is no pressure to keep costs down. Acupuncturists presently cannot get away with charging as much as medical doctors do—patients simply wouldn't pay it. But if insurance started to cover alternative medicine too (as many alternative proponents demand), the cost of alternative treatment would surely skyrocket.

Another important factor makes conventional medicine expensive: tests to "rule out" serious diseases. I frequently hear statements such as: "The M.D. put me through a battery of expensive tests, which didn't help a bit. Then I went to a chiropractor [or nutritionist, acupuncturist, Rolfer] and she cured me for half the price."

This common complaint shows a lack of appreciation of the purpose of testing. The main purpose of medical testing is to rule out serious but relatively unlikely possibilities. This can be a very useful service, but it does not by itself alleviate any symptoms.

Rolfers, acupuncturists, and chiropractors do not provide the same service. Unless they order precisely the same tests, alternative practitioners cannot rule out brain tumors, ruptured disks, fractured vertebrae, or stenosis of the spine. It isn't fair to compare the costs of medical testing against those of alternative treatment. They are different services.

The appropriate comparison would be between medical treatment and alternative treatment, leaving tests out of the equation. In the case of neck pain, medical (nonsurgical) treatment might be cheaper than chiropractic, but probably far less effective.

Another unrealistic argument states that alternative medicine is cost-effective because it prevents illnesses. I wish this were so. Unfortunately, as described in the previous section on preventive medicine, significant prevention depends more on the patient than on the doctor.

Therefore, don't expect to necessarily save money by choosing alternative treatment. You may become healthier by that choice, but that is a separate issue.

CLAIM: **Alternative Medicine Works Much Better Than Conventional Medicine.**

ANALYSIS: Proponents of alternative medicine generally believe not only that their favorite methods offer a completely different approach from that of conventional medicine, but that they are much more effective as well.

Sometimes this proposition proves true. For many conditions, alternative medicine is the best option. This is certainly the case for most conditions of chronic musculoskeletal pain; it is also true for many diseases involving subjective symptoms such as fatigue and mental confusion.

Alternative techniques can also succeed in diseases where the symptoms are not subtle at all. I remember a patient with a severe inflammation of the tissue around her heart, a condition called cardiomyopathy. It has no known cause, but it can lead to an early death. In her case, medical treatment involved seven medications, a pacemaker, and multiple trips to the hospital.

Personally, I lack the chutzpah to send a patient with such a serious disease for alternative treatment, but in this case I didn't have to—she sent herself. Working with a highly skilled Chinese herbalist, she not only managed to get off of her medications, she also reversed the cardiomyopathy itself, a result I would not have anticipated.

Testimonials such as these are thrilling to read but, unfortunately, their predictive value is limited. One success does not guarantee that any more will follow. I talked to the herbalist, and she admitted that she rarely succeeded with cardiomyopathy. In this patient's case, it was just good fortune. Nonetheless, stories like these make the rounds and lead some people to believe that alternative medicine has conventional treatment entirely beat; that medical doctors should close up their offices and go home.

Of course, such a proposal is absurd. One reason is that alternative practitioners all disagree with one another. Therefore, alternative medicine cannot be seen as a coherent replacement for conventional treatment. Also, conventional medicine has its wonderful testimonials too. Success stories abound in all healing methods—as do stories of terrible failures. No form of healing is spared disastrous outcomes. Medical doctors have been known to amputate the wrong leg, but alternative practitioners have diagnosed spinal meningitis as food allergies. The latter horror happened in Florida. It didn't make the newspapers, because the family managed to keep the error a secret out of loyalty to their elderly naturopath. But their child nearly died.

Apart from dramatic incidents such as these, it is a fact of life in alternative medicine that many patients do not get better. Chiropractic doesn't always cure neck pain, by any means, nor does acupuncture; naturopathy often fails to alleviate chronic fatigue; and homeopathy seldom succeeds with asthma. Curing illness is just plain difficult, and no doctor's success rate, no matter what method is used, approaches anywhere near 100 percent. For severe health problems, 10 or 20 percent is more likely.

Enemies and supporters of alternative medicine naturally pick and choose their stories. In reality, testimonials mean little more than that successes and failures do occur—a fact that should have been obvious from the start.

I have seen and heard of wonderful cures through every kind of treatment imaginable. Perhaps the weirdest remedy that I know of is gasoline water. Apparently, it is a custom in rural Turkey to pour water into empty gasoline cans and use the resulting broth as a medicine. A Turkish spiritual leader visiting Stanford University said that gasoline water had cured his mother's terminal cancer, and I believe him. The world of healing is mysterious. It follows its own rules and cannot be forced to follow any simple set of principles. However, I have not recommended that any of my patients concoct their own gasoline brew.

Startling anecdotes, unfortunately, say nothing about success rates. A method may work very well for one person, but only for that one out of a hundred. This is another fact of life in alternative medicine. Just because coenzyme Q10 or Rolfing cures one person's asthma (both of which I have seen), it doesn't mean the same method will work with anyone else. Many treatment methods seem reluctant to provide encore performances.

True success rates are very difficult to determine. In conventional medicine this problem is addressed through the use of controlled studies. The same method cannot be applied easily to alternative techniques. It is difficult to fit healing crafts into research models.

Proper controlled experiments should be "double-blinded." This means that neither patient nor doctor knows who is receiving real treatment, and who is getting only placebo treatment. Thus, they are both "blind."

Pills are ideally suited for double-blind experiments, for it is easy to design placebo pills that look exactly like the real medication. Neither the doctor dispensing the pills nor the patient receiving them can tell if they are real. Only the committee in charge of the experiment knows which is which.

Precautions like these are necessary to eliminate the placebo effect. If doctors knew they were dispensing fake pills, they might unwittingly communicate a lack of confidence to their patients. In double-blind experiments, doctors don't know whether the tablets they dispense are real or not. Therefore, they cannot put a positive or negative spin on the treatment.

While such experiments can easily be performed for drugs (or food supplements), double-blind studies are very difficult to perform when the treatment is a healing art like acupuncture. It is hard enough to imagine patients not knowing whether they were receiving acupuncture. But how could the acupuncturists fail to know whether or not they were providing it? (A medical acupuncturist has actually tackled this question. His research and its results are described later in this chapter.)

Many alternative practitioners with whom I have spoken discount the need for research. They feel morally certain that their methods work. Such gut feelings, however, are not reliable. Wishful thinking is a universal human trait, and practitioners of alternative medicine are no exception. Without research results, true effectiveness rates are very difficult to obtain. Until these are available, those who seek alternative treatment must rely on common sense, practical experience, and informed referrals.

CLAIM: Alternative Practitioners Know Exactly What They Are Doing.

ANALYSIS: People often form exaggerated opinions of healers. I remember Dr. Sable (not his real name), a nutritionist who traveled from city to city curing through the use of diets and food supplements. Over several years I came to know him fairly well, and discovered that he was not a flake.

Sable was motivated by a genuine desire to help people. In private he reminisced about his successes and the good feelings those gave him, rather than about his wealth (unlike some other successful healers I have known). Diligent, thoughtful, and always studying, he was one of the finest traveling nutritionists I have met. I frequently referred patients to him.

Nonetheless, he was not the demigod his patients made him out to be. According to the cult of Sable, he could cure anything, and had—you name it: cancer, multiple sclerosis, bad breath. There was no limit to his powers. His patients imagined that he was privy to some extraordinarily complex system of healing, but I knew from speaking to him that Sable's methods were not profound. He had a bag of tricks and simply tried them all.

All good healers are idealized by patients with whom they have succeeded. Even I have been the victim of such excessive admiration. Unfortunately, it is just a fantasy. No healer of any persuasion knows very much about health and illness. None ever know exactly what they are doing, and very often they are completely in the dark. The world of ignorance dwarfs the world of knowledge, by far.

Having analyzed some claims alternative medicine advocates make on their own behalf, I will now turn to criticisms coming from outside. The following four propositions are widely believed by medical doctors.

CLAIM: Alternative Practitioners Are Quacks Who Keep Patients Away from Responsible Treatment.

ANALYSIS: According to this widely held view, alternative practitioners are menaces to the public health. They are fools at best, crooks at worst, always ready to snatch insulin syringes from the hands of diabetic youngsters in favor of chamomile tea. This paranoid fantasy is the equivalent in reverse of what many alternative proponents think about the conventional medical profession.

Alternative and conventional practitioners tend to dislike and demonize one another. Fortunately, the real world is not so easily divided into heroes and villains. Alternative medicine, like any other field, attracts practitioners of various qualities. I have known many whose integrity would be remarkable anywhere, and a few whose insincerity and avarice would shock a used-car salesman.

Medical doctors who believe all alternative practitioners are quacks simply have never gotten to know a good one personally. (They generally move in different social circles.) Ignorance supports stereotyping. I have worked with dozens of alternative therapists whose pragmatism, intelligence, honesty, effort, and humility have impressed me deeply. Later in the book, I describe several of these worthy physicians and healers.

The majority of alternative practitioners believe what they preach to others, and put into practice most of their own beliefs. Of course, sincerity does not guarantee correctness, but it does cut down on con artistry. Few alternative therapists are outright cheats.

Unconscious commercialism, however, is a common problem. For example, many alternative providers are in the habit of earning a little extra income by selling food supplements. This practice is rationalized as "making the highest-quality products available to clients." But, human nature being what it is, when there is a profit to be gained by it, more supplements will be sold.

Selling what one prescribes is a conflict of interest; it has a corrupting effect. Imagine what would happen if doctors sold medications: how alternative practitioners would howl! Alternative providers who sell food supplements are just as liable to rightful critique. Of course, many do so with full integrity, but the mere appearance of conflicting interests lowers professional standards.

There are other examples of institutional commercialism in alternative medicine. Routine weekly visits to the chiropractor or the acupuncturist are seldom terminated by the practitioners. There always seems to be a reason for another visit. Of course, medical doctors enjoy similar benefits. I have heard many internists gloat over patients whose medical condition mandates frequent visits; similarly, neurologists salivate over routine nerve-conduction studies. Healing, after all, is a job. It is impossible to eliminate financial motivation entirely.

The proposition heading this section makes a second charge besides quackery: it states that alternative practitioners keep patients away from responsible treatment. This probably did occur with some frequency in the past. The public was more credulous then, and much less well informed. In my experience, modern alternative practitioners seldom counsel their patients to throw their drugs away or avoid life-saving surgery. They do not do so for one simple reason: they are afraid to. Alternative therapists are just as terrified of lawsuits as anyone else. Few alternative practitioners (besides chiropractors) have malpractice insurance. A civil action would be catastrophic. Also, the fierce vigilance with which medical boards prosecute alternative practitioners keeps most of them chastened and on guard.

Most licensed alternative practitioners are taught to avoid direct conflict with standard medical practice. Acupuncturists, for example, learn to be diplomatic and to work congenially with their patients' physicians. Typically, alternative practitioners encourage their patients to use their own common sense, and to taper off their dosage of drugs (for example) only if decreasing symptoms allow it and their doctors concur.

Besides the relatively mild attitudes of modern alternative practitioners, health consumers themselves have matured tremendously in recent decades. Most people seem to be able to make up their own minds quite responsibly as to which situations require conventional medical intervention and which do not.

CLAIM: Alternative Medicine Is Nothing but Snake Oil, Superstition, and Fantasy.

ANALYSIS: This accusation is partly true: alternative medicine is brimming over with inaccuracy, nonsense, and groundless beliefs. However, the field also embodies much that is correct, valuable, and even profound.

Unfortunately, the valuable and worthless aspects of alternative medicine are mixed together as closely as the particles in homogenized milk. Insufficient research makes it very difficult to distinguish between useful methods and wistful dreams. When seeking help from alternative practitioners, patients must rely heavily on their own intelligence and discrimination and pay close attention to actual results.

Some types of alternative medicine may be trusted more than others. As a general rule, methods that have withstood the test of time are more dependable than fads. Therefore, acupuncture may be expected to succeed more often than the favorite cure-all of a particular season.

Treatment methods of less historical lineage possess correspondingly greater amounts of pure tripe. Faddish ideas are often passed by word of mouth and from book to book, without the benefit of any intervening critical thinking, actual clinical experience, or solid research. More than once I have been tempted to give up on alternative medicine entirely because of its nonsense, only to be drawn back by some deep skill or remarkable success.

Alternative medicine supports high levels of foolishness because it isn't scientific. For all its flaws, science possesses excellent methods for discriminating reality from fiction. This filter is sorely missed in alternative healing.

In order to achieve reliability, however, scientists have to ignore everything that can't be quantified. This leaves out many good options. In real life, many worthwhile goals are achieved without the benefit of a team of researchers. Finish carpentry is not a pie-in-the-sky dream simply because it isn't based on academic experimentation; nor has Ming dynasty ceramic ware been outclassed by the products of modern factories. A person who pursues a goal with integrity, skill, common sense, and close attention can often succeed without the benefit of formal methods.

This is precisely what occurs in alternative medicine. The higher forms of alternative medicine are informed by a depth and caring that make their results meaningful. For example, Chinese acupuncturists of past centuries paid close attention to the results of their interventions. When certain methods didn't work, they changed course and experimented until they found a way to succeed. Pragmatic efforts such as these deserve respect. Although they are not as reproducible as the products of medical science, they are much more than superstition, fantasy, or snake oil.

It should also be pointed out that many widely used conventional treatments are unproved as well. These include, for starters: antibiotic therapy for colds, epidural steroid injections for back pain, physical therapy for neck pain, and intravenous corticosteroids for shock. By some estimates, only 15 percent of conventional medicine is fully scientific. Bear in mind, however, this is a lot higher percentage than can be found in any aspect of alternative medicine.

CLAIM: Alternative Medicine Is All Placebo
(Power of Suggestion).

ANALYSIS: Some physicians are willing to concede that alternative practitioners may be honest, and admit that alternative medicine sometimes succeeds. However, they attribute all these successes to the placebo effect. In their opinion, the only reason any alternative technique works is that through warmth of personality and the power of suggestion, practitioners cause their patients to expect improvement.

This gracious explanation is actually an insult. It trivializes alternative medicine and characterizes as mere self-hypnosis all the efforts alternative practitioners undergo to master their chosen arts. Even Andrew Weil appears to believe that it is primarily the alternative practitioner's belief in his or her method, rather than its independent efficacy, that serves to heal.

No doubt the power of suggestion plays a role in all healing interactions. But to say that alternative medicine is no more than placebo is to make a sweeping judgment that is not justified by the facts. It is absurd to believe that none of the sincere practitioners of alternative medicine have ever discovered any useful techniques. To presume this is to engage in a kind of peculiar religious faith, the belief that medical science encompasses all that anyone knows about healing. This is not a rational belief.

In fact, the placebo explanation can be soundly refuted on several grounds. First, there is the evidence of numerous controlled studies. Alternative medicine is relatively weak in the area of research, but plenty of good research does exist; there simply have not been enough completed studies to give alternative medicine anything like a comprehensive scientific foundation. However, far more than enough has been done to disprove the universal placebo hypothesis. For one startling example, acupuncture as a treatment for dysmenorrhea has been evaluated by controlled experiment. The results show that acupuncture does relieve menstrual pain.

Acupuncture is practically impossible to fit into the standard double-blind experimental model. Nonetheless, this feat has been accomplished by Joseph Helms, M.D., in a yearlong research study conducted in Oakland, California.

To make it possible, he used a simplified form of acupuncture. Several technicians were trained to insert needles in certain points that are generally useful for menstrual pain. Unbeknownst to the technicians, some were given information sheets containing the wrong point locations. The instructors did not see the sheets and, therefore, did not know which of their students were being deceived. All the trainees believed that they were performing real acupuncture, but only half of them really were. The patients who were to be treated by these technicians were divided into two corresponding groups, secretly called "the real acupuncture group" and "the placebo acupuncture group."

In fact, acupuncture that is standardized to a fixed set of points is an inferior form of the art. True acupuncture is highly individualized. However, all the acupuncture used in this experiment was artificially standardized as described, in order to fit it into the double-blind model.

Despite the fact that this was second-rate acupuncture treatment, the real acupuncture group suffered far less menstrual pain than the placebo acupuncture group. Both groups received identical levels of attention from treaters fully confident that they were performing effective treatment. The fact that one group experienced fewer symptoms is strong evidence that more than a placebo effect was at work.

Thousands more good studies exist, especially in the field of food supplement therapy. Besides the evidence of formal research, daily clinical practice also shows that alternative medicine can be far more than a placebo. Emma Seabright is a typical example. Before she came to me, she had suffered from severe migraine headaches more than twice a week for twenty years. Emma had tried all the available migraine medications, as well as chiropractic, food supplement therapy, and Western herbology. Nothing worked well. Migraines continued to make her life miserable.

After thirty sessions of acupuncture, her headaches disappeared entirely, and remained absent for the several more years I continued to know her. Of course, acupuncture treatment doesn't always work this well. The point of this story is not the superiority of acupuncture over other modalities. What I am trying to say is that Emma's experience, like so many other patients' I have seen, disproves the placebo theory. If acupuncture treatment was only a placebo, why hadn't all her other treatments served as a placebo too?

In my opinion, the placebo effect is real, but its effects are limited. Many people who suffer from chronic pain, for example, respond for a week or two to almost any new treatment, but the effect does not last. The mind easily accepts suggestions, but it apparently cannot hold them for very long. As time passes, the suggestive effect wears off, and the symptom returns. Therefore, placebo methods are much more useful for acute conditions than for chronic ones. Conversely, when the effects of a treatment last for many months, it is unrealistic to attribute them to the placebo effect.

One last objection to the placebo theory is this: If placebo were the primary factor in every alternative treatment, believers should do significantly better than nonbelievers. This has not been my experience. I have seen many nonbelievers cured, while numerous believers walk away dissatisfied.

Alternative medicine, like all forms of medicine, involves a mixture of suggestion and effects that are independent of suggestion. In other words, many alternative techniques work objectively.

CLAIM: Alternative Treatments Are Dangerous.

ANALYSIS: This statement, although often repeated, is plainly incorrect. Nearly all alternative medical techniques are far safer than those promoted by conventional medicine.

I once aroused a storm of controversy by saying this in my newspaper column. Thinking it a rather self-evident remark, I wrote, "To some extent, all drugs are poisonous." Actually, my remark was a watered-down version of what a pharmacology professor at my medical school had taught. His exact words were: "All drugs are poisons." I thought my statement rather mild in comparison.

With few exceptions, most pharmaceuticals could serve as excellent replacements for arsenic in murder mysteries. The point in my column was not to demonize drugs, however. I believe that life involves compromises, and that in many situations a medication may be the best option. Rather, I meant to emphasize that drugs are not the equivalent of bran muffins or broccoli, and they should not be used when there are other good options.

The local medical community took strenuous exception to my remarks. One physician screamed at me over the phone, "Patients will read your column, think their drugs are poisons, stop taking them and die! It will be your fault!" The president of the local medical society felt compelled to write a rebuttal to my column. In it, he stated that many substances are poisonous if used incorrectly, even vitamins and herbs.

While this is literally true, it is substantially misleading. There is a huge difference in magnitude between the toxicity of pharmaceuticals and that of vitamins. To prove this, I have proposed the following dare to anyone who believes vitamins are just as dangerous as drugs: Let us both be blindfolded. I will be placed in a health food store, you behind the counter at a pharmacy. We will each select a bottle at random, and remove our blindfolds. Each of us will then take ten times the recommended daily dose of whatever substance we hold in our hands.

Obviously, no sane person would take such a dare. There are few substances in a health food store that would do more than give me a stomachache if I took ten times the recommended dose; anyone who similarly tried his or her luck in a pharmacy would be fortunate to walk out alive.

Not only are health food remedies safer than drugs, natural treatment techniques such as massage and chiropractic are far more benign than surgeries and epidural steroid injections. Of course, one can find occasional horror stories, but they are rare and, as mentioned earlier, they may be found on both sides of the aisle.

As a practical matter, the worst danger of alternative treatment is the real possibility that it may not work, and you may waste your money.

The best way to utilize any service is to perceive its strengths and weaknesses accurately. Clearly, broad generalizations about alternative medicine, whether positive or negative, do not reflect reality. It is therefore important to cut through the rhetoric and pay careful attention to the actual nature of this diverse and extensive field.

SECTION II

SCIENTIFIC APPROACHES TO HEALING

Alternative medicine comes in two flavors: methods that attempt to achieve a scientific approach to healing, and others that are better described as crafts. This section deals with the first category.

Most doctors would say that conventional medicine is truly scientific and alternative medicine is unscientific, but it isn't that simple. The naturopathic branch of alternative medicine in particular is increasingly scientific in its orientation, while the science in conventional medicine remains far from complete.

The question of the scientific validity of alternative therapies came to the forefront in Washington State in late 1995. As part of its attempts at health care reform, the Washington legislature passed a law requiring insurance companies to pay for alternative practitioners. The state's insurance companies weren't too happy about this, and dragged their feet. Then, Washington's activist insurance commissioner Deborah Senn took action. She issued bulletins ordering insurance companies to cover alternative practitioners under most health insurance policies they sold.

When this became known, the public responded with wild enthusiasm. I personally received a flood of calls inquiring about new options, and Senn's office held a series of public meetings to explain what was happening. The attendance and media exposure were remarkable. A spirit of revolutionary change could be felt in the air.

Under this pressure, the major insurers began holding meetings with alternative care providers to set standards for treatment and to work out other necessary arrangements. For a few months, it looked as if acupuncturists, massage thera-pists, chiropractors, and naturopaths would be receiving insurance coverage by early 1996.

Then came the backlash. About four months after the law was passed, the state's largest insurance companies filed suit to block implementation of the regu-lations. The lawsuit itself was based on a number of technical points, but the companies' real complaint was this: under the new law, they felt they would be forced to cover unscientific methods that had never been proved to work. "What if these treatments hurt people?" one insurance executive asked me. "What if they are a complete waste of time? I'm all for alternative medicine, but only if it has been scientifically evaluated and proved cost-effective."

Incensed by their sudden change of fortunes, alternative providers counterat-tacked, claiming that conventional medicine is not wholly scientific either. "Many medical treatments have not been proved effective either," they said. "Why should those methods be covered, when ours are not?"

It was a good question. As I write this, the matter is still unresolved. Perhaps a judge ultimately will have to determine what is truly scientific and what is not, and whether only scientific forms of treatment should be covered by insurance. But such a legal battle would only be one part of a larger debate regarding the relationship between science and healing.

WHAT IS A SCIENTIFIC APPROACH TO HEALING?

A scientific approach to anything involves standardized methods, detailed investi-gation into how they work, and precise measurements of the results of applying them. Conventional medicine attempts to function in this way, and succeeds to a greater extent than has any other approach to healing. However, the job of making medicine completely scientific is still far from complete. The alternative practition-ers' complaints were correct. According to experts at Duke University, only about 15 percent of medical interventions are supported by solid scientific evidence.

For example, while there is no question that antibiotics can speed up the healing of individual ear infections, most doctors will also say that antibiotic treatment is necessary to prevent complications such as hearing loss and meningitis. But in fact, no good evidence proves that the routine treatment of ear infections actually prevents any of these complications. Some European studies suggest that *not* treating ear infections gives better results overall. Nonetheless, conventional physicians always prescribe antibiotics for ear infections in this country. It is really just a custom.

One of the medical directors at a large health maintenance organization (HMO) told me confidentially that his company wanted to stop treating ear infections. "We believe in evidence-based medicine here," he said. "But there is no evidence that children need to take amoxicillin every time their eardrums are red." He went on to say, however, that his company did not dare to stop treating ear infections. "It would get in the newspapers. We'd be tarred and feathered for depriving children of treatment," he said—depriving them of treatment they don't really need!

Much of modern conventional medicine consists simply of tradition, habit, and unproved reasoning—just like its alternative counterparts. Nonetheless, there is a difference in degree. Conventional medicine is a thousand times more scientific than most branches of alternative medicine. Acupuncture can point to no more than a couple dozen good studies on it's behalf. The only form of alternative treatment that comes remotely near the level of science in conventional medicine is modern naturopathic medicine.

Naturopathy is described in detail later in this section. It consists mainly of diet, food supplements, and herbs. In a way, this field can be considered a younger cousin of conventional medicine, with many similarities.

Like conventional medicine with its leeches, naturopathy began as a thoroughly unscientific approach to healing. The original naturopaths of the 1800s based their treatments mostly on a passion for "getting back to nature." But in the last quarter century naturopathy has increasingly adopted scientific attitudes and methodologies. Naturopathy today is based to a great extent on biological research.

For example, a standardized extract of the herb black cohosh (used for menopausal symptoms) has been evaluated in controlled trials involving more than a hundred women. This number is still low by conventional medical standards, but it's nothing to sneeze at. Even with the limited funding available to it, naturopathy is making a serious attempt to ground itself in solid science. For this it deserves respect.

Unfortunately, some of the references cited in books on alternative medicine involve testing on no more than a handful of people. For example, Dr. Julian Whitaker in his *Guide to Natural Healing* says that "L-tyrosine has been shown as effective as anti-depressant drugs [in the treatment of depression]." A footnote refers to Melvyn Werbach's *Nutritional Influences on Mental Illness.*

I looked up the footnote. According to Werbach, the best study of L-tyrosine for depression involved only five people who took the supplement. Three of them showed improvement after four weeks. While one must suppose that those three patients were grateful for feeling better, a sample size of five simply doesn't prove much.

The following diagram roughly estimates the level of science in these two forms of medicine. Notice that naturopathic and conventional medicine overlap each other, but naturopathic medicine leans farther toward the unscientific end of the scale than does conventional medicine.

Comparative level of science in naturopathic medicine and conventional medicine.

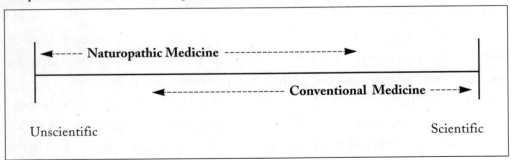

The chapters of this section address the most important partially scientific approaches to healing. In the years to come, further study will continue to separate the worthwhile from the worthless in these fields. Scientific validation will in turn lead to increased mainstream acceptability; ultimately, what proves valid among the alternative methods discussed in this section will likely become part of conventional treatment.

CHAPTER 3

Conventional Medicine

It may seem peculiar to discuss conventional medicine in a book about alternative treatments, but conventional medicine is simply one alternative among many. It is the most widely used, to be sure, and the one with the most power and authority. For many Americans, however, it is only one option, and not necessarily the first one to be tried.

In other countries, Western medicine (as it is called) is even more obviously optional. I have a friend from the Punjab region of India who tells me that medical clinics there typically have three entrances. One door leads to a practitioner of Ayurveda, the traditional medicine of India. Another opens on the office of a homeopath. The third door leads to a Western-trained medical doctor. People choose which practitioner to go to based on what problem they are suffering from. For broken bones, asthma, severe infections, and high blood pressure, my friend and his family would visit the Western doctor. For stomach problems, headaches, sinus allergies, and colds they might choose the Ayurvedic practitioner. And for chronic problems like skin diseases, depression, and arthritis they might try the homeopath. If one physician failed, they would try another.

We may be moving toward a day where a similar spectrum of choices will be available in this country. The advantage of having such a choice is that each form of healing has its own characteristic strengths and weaknesses and can complement the others.

Conventional medicine approaches the body as if it were a complex machine, and seeks to develop and refine treatments by understanding the workings of that machine. As we all know, this biomechanical approach can be very successful. Medical researchers have developed powerful and effective treatments for a wide variety of acute and chronic illnesses.

But the mechanical orientation of conventional medicine causes problems too. Not the least of these is the loss of a human touch. Indeed, this is one of the reasons more people are turning to alternative approaches. Medical treatments can be harsh, humiliating, and invasive. And the tools and philosophies of conventional medicine have had an effect on physicians themselves: medical doctors are becoming progressively more like engineers and less like warm, empathic caregivers. As one of my patients said, "My doctor looks at me as if I were a broken appliance."

Doctors are typically more excited by the discovery of rare and unusual conditions than the daily process of helping people in need. Many have lost awareness of the softer side of life and instead see only statistics and technology. Their training leads them to instinctively dislike "simple natural remedies," and to automatically prefer high-tech interventions.

This is not intended as a criticism—it is merely a description. However, the medical profession does deserve critique on one count at least: its belief that conventional medicine alone possesses everything that is to be known about healing. This dogma is patently absurd. Of all the millions of people throughout history who have sought to heal illnesses, some must have discovered useful information. Conventional medicine cannot possibly hold a monopoly on knowledge.

It is true that modern medicine's knowledge is the most solidly *validated*. The methods of conventional medicine have been more fully studied than those of any alternative technique. More so than with chiropractic, acupuncture, or naturopathy, you know what you are getting with conventional medicine.

But in order to make sure of its findings, conventional medicine has had to concentrate its attention on what can be studied easily. This mostly means pills. All approaches that could not be measured and standardized have been disregarded as being too "fuzzy." This category includes all the subtly sophisticated, subjective, and intuitive methods used by the many healing arts. Many of these "soft" approaches can sometimes treat problems that resist the rigid methods of scientific medicine.

THE LIMITATIONS OF CONVENTIONAL MEDICINE

I often encounter patients who prefer alternative medicine but must occasionally interact with conventional doctors. To them I make the following suggestion: Be sure to adjust your expectations to reality. Realize that medical doctors have sharply limited powers.

For example, it is not appropriate to expect medical doctors to be sensitive healers. The modern doctor is largely limited to the role of biomechanical engineer. Understanding this will forestall disappointment.

Another important point is that doctors do not actually pay attention to everything they hear. While they are definitely interested in facts, only facts that pertain to a known diagnosis hold their attention. When doctors hear certain important key phrases, such as "crushing chest pain" or "a strange change in this mole," they take note. But symptoms that don't fit any known picture seem extraneous, and doctors will ignore them. In fact, there is no reason for them to pay attention. Even if they were all ears, it wouldn't make any difference. A medical doctor simply cannot do anything about symptoms that don't fit into a known pattern.

Patients are often unaware of this and get their feelings hurt. I remember a woman who was infuriated because, no matter how often she complained about it, her doctor ignored her complaints of excessive daytime sweating. I explained that he did so because excessive daytime sweating is not a symptom of any disease she was likely to have. Therefore, there was nothing the doctor could do with the information. He should have told her so politely, but medical doctors are sometimes not the greatest communicators.

Other limitations of conventional medicine are also worth recognizing. For example, although not many people realize it, there are thousands of conditions for which the best efforts of conventional medicine are largely ineffective. The most obvious of these is chronic soft-tissue pain. Conventional medicine is practically useless for conditions such as neck and back pain. Medical doctors know this, but because they do not countenance the many useful alternative options available (such as chiropractic and acupuncture), they feel inadequate when patients come to them with these problems. Out of this sense of frustration comes the unfortunate dismissal, "It must be all in your head." This infamous phrase is seldom an instance of deep psychological perception. Most often it is really a confession of helplessness.

Besides health problems for which there is no effective conventional treatment, many other ailments do have treatments, but at a cost in side effects that may not be worthwhile.

Finally, there are many vague conditions with which medicine cannot come to grips at all. This category includes such conditions as environmental illness, fibromyalgia, food allergies, chronic fatigue syndrome, low resistance to illness, general "unwellness," and many others.

I recommend that patients try to avoid getting angry at medical doctors when they fail to help. It is important to remember that physicians are not gods. They have a limited set of tools available for their use. Either there is a known medical treatment available or there is not. If there is a treatment, but it produces very unpleasant side effects, doctors may simply have nothing else to try.

Fortunately, there are often good alternative treatments to be found when conventional medicine falls short.

CHAPTER 4

Naturopathic Medicine

Most people have never heard of naturopathy by name. Its methods, however, are among the most famous and popular forms of alternative medicine. Just about everything sold in health food stores belongs to the naturopathic tradition, and virtually all the writing available on natural foods, diet, and natural healing originates in the naturopathic thinking of the past two centuries. Juicing, fasting, colonic irrigation, drinking a gallon of water a day, "proper" food combining, raw foods theory, vegetarianism, herbal medicine, and (more recently) vitamins and food supplements were all made popular in America by naturopathic practitioners.

Naturopathy is a separate profession in only a few states, where it is practiced by N.D.s, or naturopaths. But the general methods traditionally associated with naturopathy are used by a variety of practitioners. Most M.D.s who define themselves as "alternative" or "holistic" practice variations on the theme of naturopathy, and when chiropractors, nutritionists, holistic nurses, and massage therapists recommend food supplements or herbs, they too are functioning as de facto naturopaths.

In the past twenty-five years or so, naturopathy has involved itself to an increasing extent with biochemistry, scientific research, and treatments that come in pills. It is fair to say that next to conventional medicine, modern naturopathic medicine is the most scientific of all approaches to healing. But it was not always this way. In its original nineteenth-century form, naturopathy was primarily an emotional and spiritual phenomenon, an important part of the first wave of the back-to-nature movement. It is important to consider this history, for even the most scientific aspects of naturopathy today are still colored by these nonscientific influences. Also, some naturopathic practitioners passionately resist the "scientificization" of naturopathic medicine, considering it a kind of sellout.

THE ORIGINS OF NATUROPATHY

It is impossible to trace an exact beginning to the movement that spawned naturopathy, but Jean Jacques Rousseau (1712–1778) was certainly one of the first prominent writers to popularize back-to-nature ideals. His criticism of the filth of the newly industrializing cities and his praiseful regard for "the state of nature" had a tremendous influence both in Europe and in America.

Subsequently, a new philosophy of healing was born: the belief that the key to restoring health lay in returning humans to their "natural state." Many of the first advocates of the "nature cure" lived in Germany. At a time when medical doctors were poisoning their patients with mercury and bleeding them to death, doctors such as Vincent Preissnitz (1799–1851) advocated curing patients by taking them on walks into the woods, meadows, and along wild rivers. Other German "nature doctors" emphasized fasting, simple diet, and the healing powers of fresh air and sunlight. Father Sebastian Kneipp (1821–1897) recommended "taking the water-cure" in natural hot springs.

America made a contribution to early naturopathy as well. Thomsonianism was an influential American system of herbal treatment that flourished in the early 1800s. Another school, the Hygienic movement, was co-founded by Sylvester Graham (of "graham cracker" fame). It advocated vegetarianism and the use of whole grains. Yet another famous name was John Harvey Kellogg (the founder of Kellogg's cereal), who stressed the dangers of constipation.

These practitioners regarded conventional medicine as the enemy of health. They recognized in medicine's nascent scientific thrust a desire to "improve on nature" by artificial means. They saw this goal as fundamentally wrongheaded.

Benedict Lust (1869–1945) was the first to popularize the word *naturopath*. A German immigrant and disciple of Father Kneipp, he worked tirelessly to promote the "Naturopathic school of medicine." He also founded the world's first health food store in New York City. Other writers and healers followed his lead, including such notables as Jethro Kloss and Gaylord Hauser.

From 1920 to the beginnings of World War II, naturopathic medicine flourished as a popular alternative to conventional medicine. It emphasized restoring *wellness* to the *whole person* through *natural means*—a goal that encompasses the three great ideals of alternative medicine.

The increasingly powerful AMA constantly attempted to destroy what it viewed as quackery. Professional competition no doubt played a role, but more importantly, medical doctors were on a campaign to make the world a more "scientific" place. They viewed the back-to-nature ideal as superstitious romanticism and an obstacle to progress.

Conventional medicine intended to improve on nature through science and technology. But naturopaths opposed chemicals, even going so far as to claim that chemicals used in agriculture could cause cancer (a radical concept at the time). This was not what medical doctors wanted to hear. They viewed chemicals as the best source of new medical treatments and expected great medical advances to flow from the developing science of biochemistry.

Benedict Lust and others fought a vigorous and continuous battle to defend naturopathy against the AMA's attacks. But with the discovery of sulfa and penicillin, and the death of Lust in 1945, naturopathy in America began to decline. In state after state, naturopathic practitioners were hounded from practice in a systematic campaign of persecution that bears a resemblance to the McCarthy era Red scare. "Unscientific" was next to "un-American" as a term of condemnation. Perhaps motivated by a genuine desire to rid the world of "snake oil," as well as for less noble reasons, by the 1950s the AMA had bullied naturopathy out of the public arena. It was not to reemerge as a significant force for more than twenty years.

NATUROPATHIC CONCEPTS AND THEORIES

Besides the general principle of returning to nature, several specific approaches have become characteristic of naturopathy. While practitioners and patients often assume that the following concepts are solidly established universal medical truths, they actually belong specifically to the naturopathic tradition. None are accepted by conventional practitioners, nor are they universally believed by practitioners of all branches of alternative medicine. Traditional Chinese medicine, for example, disagrees with many staple naturopathic theories.

The Need for Detoxification

The first and one of the most famous principles of naturopathy is the approach to treatment called detoxification. This concept originated in the intuitions of the early naturopaths. Observing the unhealthy lifestyle habits and polluted surroundings of their contemporaries, these physicians concluded that much illness was caused by toxic pollution. In this perception they were far ahead of their time, anticipating many of the concerns of the modern environmental sciences.

Naturopathic concern over toxicity developed into a global philosophy of illness. Illnesses were understood as releases of toxins. Stored toxins were thought to reside in body fat, to be released during periods of weight loss. Meat, fermented food, and coffee, among other substances, were supposed to produce internal putrefaction and poisoning. Constipation was said by Kellogg to cause "autointoxication" and to lie at the root of many illnesses.

Toxicity became almost the physical equivalent of evil, and a host of purgative practices were developed to detoxify the body. These included flushing the kidneys by drinking copious amounts of water, inducing the liver to release toxic buildup by means of the "liver flush" and coffee enemas, causing the skin to sweat poisons by means of juice fasts and saunas, and emptying the colon through high enemas and lower-bowel tonics.

While it is scientifically clear that the kidney, liver, and intestines do remove toxins in the ordinary course of their activities, there is no objective evidence of any health benefits to be gained by the special efforts described in the preceding paragraph. Their use is mainly based on naturopathic intuitions. For this reason, conventional medicine rejects these methods.

Furthermore, some of the classic detoxification techniques are obviously founded on false beliefs. For example, it has long been a widely held view among naturopathically inclined practitioners that most people's colons are caked with layer upon layer of deposited toxins. These toxins are supposedly set down like sedimentary rock from the accumulation of decades of poor diet. Whole books have been written (and are still being written) on "colon cleansing," which may involve high enemas, juice fasting, psyllium husks and flaxseed, and many other steps to peel away the accumulated poisons.

However, medical doctors have been performing regular examinations of the colon to look for bowel cancer for the last twenty years or more. Most of these patients are at least middle-aged. According to the theory, they should possess extremely toxic colons. Upon examination, however, none prove to have any coating on the fresh pink flesh of the colon. There is no black residue, no thick deposits, no indication of toxins in the colon. The theory of colonic layering has thus been proved wrong. Strangely, no one in the alternative health movement appears to have paid attention. The old description of caked colons continues.

Despite the fact that the principle on which it is based is incorrect, colon cleansing does sometimes produce significant health benefits. I remember a patient who apparently cured herself of chronic sinus infections solely through colonics. This is the same phenomenon alluded to many times in this book: alternative methods whose justification makes little rational sense nonetheless sometimes produce excellent results.

All the other methods of detoxification occasionally produce definite health benefits as well. Of course, it is possible that they work for some other reason having nothing to do with the concept of detoxification. But it seems to me likely that once again naturopaths have intuitively hit on an aspect of the truth.

A final note: Like every other medical approach, detoxification can sometimes be carried too far. I have seen people make themselves sick through overly exuberant attempts at self-purification.

Homeopathic Principles

Another set of beliefs commonly held by naturopathic practitioners are actually homeopathic principles. (The homeopathic school of medicine is described in more detail in the next chapter.) Homeopathic thinking was not a part of traditional naturopathy. Indeed, homeopaths and naturopaths fiercely criticized each other at first. However, three homeopathic concepts eventually took root in the practices of naturopathy: (1) If a symptom is suppressed without being cured, it will pop up elsewhere. (2) During the process of recovery, old symptoms will return in reverse order of how they were originally experienced. (3) In order to get better, a person may first have to get worse.

Conventional medicine has not observed any of these patterns. However, some alternative practitioners believe they have seen these patterns, and they regard these principles as indisputable.

The Primacy of Digestion

Another traditional current of naturopathy attributes great health significance to digestion. Many diseases are thought to be caused by inadequate digestion or by incomplete absorption of nutrients. In order to enhance digestive powers, naturopaths often suggest supplements such as bromelain, betaine hydrochloride, apple cider vinegar, pancreatic enzymes, and herbal bitters. They also may believe that high doses of vitamins and minerals are necessary to overcome malabsorption.

Another traditional naturopathic recommendation for better digestion involves rules of "proper" food combining. Most health food stores sell small laminated cards summarizing these principles. Because they are based on outdated discoveries regarding digestive physiology, I do not give them much credence.

In my experience, methods based on improving digestion and absorption can sometimes resolve serious health problems. For example, I recall a patient who successfully cured her back pain by means of pancreatic enzymes, and another who was able to stop taking asthma medications through the use of betaine hydrochloride. This is a theory that obviously has some truth to it. In real life, however, digestive aids do not produce such dramatic effects every day.

Weak Adrenals

Besides poor digestion, naturopathic alternative practitioners typically relate numerous problems to "weak adrenal glands. Like the concept of detoxification, this is a rather loose notion. Treatments aimed at strengthening the adrenals sometimes work, but whether the adrenal glands themselves actually have anything to do with the syndrome named after them is an open question.

Strengthening the Immune System

Finally, alternative practitioners inspired by naturopathy frequently speak of injury to the immune system and propose various means of restoring it.

In actuality, the immune system is not one entity. It is a collection of systems by which the body defends itself from infection. Modern scientific understanding has only penetrated a little way into this subject; much of how immunity works is little understood.

Nonetheless, many naturopathic practitioners believe that they can boost the patient's immunity. Methods intended to accomplish this may involve herbs such as echinacea, ginseng, and astragalus, or supplements such as vitamin C and whole thymus extract. These are used for many purposes, including preventing colds and other infections, treating infections once they have arisen, and minimizing the symptoms of allergies and multiple sclerosis.

Interestingly, Chinese medicine disagrees with some of the methods used by alternative practitioners to raise immunity: in particular, the indiscriminate use of ginseng and astragalus. These are Chinese herbs, and so perhaps the warnings of Chinese medical experts should be taken seriously.

According to traditional Chinese herbology, ginseng and astragalus are useful only for certain aspects of immunity. Astragalus is often used by practitioners of Chinese herbology to prevent colds. Traditional Oriental herbalists, however, believe that once a cold has begun, astragalus can make it worse. Naturopathic practitioners seldom recognize this distinction, and prescribe astragalus to everyone as a general immune tonic.

In my experience it is possible to enhance immunity, however, it is more a matter of improving balance holistically than of pumping people full of some purported immune "booster."

THE "SCIENTIFICIZATION"
OF NATUROPATHY

During the 1950s, faith in conventional medicine reached a peak never to be equaled again. The dramatic cures produced by antibiotics and the epidemic-destroying powers of the Salk polio vaccine had so impressed the public that it seemed doctors could do no wrong.

The possibility that accepted medical treatments could be dangerous or inappropriate was little suspected by anyone. Doctors used radiation therapy for such problems as sore throats and acne, never dreaming that by doing so they were causing cancer; they prescribed drugs like thalidomide and DES (diethylstilbestrol) unaware of the epidemic of birth defects to follow; and they delivered babies drugged unconscious by the anesthetic given to their mothers as if this were a great improvement over natural childbirth. Disillusionment would come later, but in the 1950s science and technology ruled supreme.

No wonder naturopathy went into decline. In such a context, no profession of healing based on repudiating conventional medicine could attract the public interest. The desire for natural treatment, however, was too powerful and enduring simply to disappear. It was soon reborn under a different and more scientific guise: as nutritional medicine.

Perhaps more than anyone else, Adelle Davis was responsible for this new approach. Her popular books taught the postwar generation to pay attention to what it ate. Diet had always been important to naturopaths. But Davis's works were different from previous naturopathic writing: they were solidly grounded in the scientific knowledge of the day and phrased in a style that was respectful of the medical establishment. This was an altogether novel approach.

Adelle Davis also popularized the use of vitamins, a method of treatment that would eventually alter the entire landscape of naturopathy. Through her influence, health food store shelves began to be increasingly stocked with vitamin pills, replacing the older packages of wheat germ, nutritional yeast, and liver extract.

Vitamins continued to grow in popularity throughout the 1960s. With the 1970 publication of Linus Pauling's *Vitamin C and the Common Cold,* vitamins positively exploded onto the national scene. From that point on, vitamins and other food supplements would be a mainstay of alternative medicine. And when naturopathy reemerged as a profession in the late 1970s, vitamin therapy and biochemical research would be dominant influences.

This was a historic change of direction. In its original form, naturopathy functioned more as a spiritual philosophy than as a scientific endeavor. To people like Father Kneipp, true healing consisted in returning to God's original plan for humanity. As in the influential book of the same name by Jethro Kloss, natural medicine wanted to take the world *Back to Eden.* "God has provided a remedy for every disease that might afflict us," Kloss wrote in his widely quoted and influential text. "Man's methods of treating disease are truly complicated and mystifying, but God's ways are so simple that anyone can understand them without a medical education. . . . The fundamental principle of true healing consists of a return to natural habits of living."

Kloss would not have approved of vitamin C. "Recently a Chicago firm advertised very extensively some little tablets," he complained, "claiming that they contained all the elements needed by the body, and were prepared by scientifically combining foods . . . [but] the most learned scientists who ever lived on this earth cannot separate natural foods and then combine them in a better manner than nature herself has prepared them."

Adelle Davis and Linus Pauling did not base their recommendations on faith in providence; they turned to science as a justification. Obviously, nature had not provided vitamin C pills to cure man's ills. Scientists had simply identified the vitamin as an important constituent of a healthy diet. Davis and Pauling did rebuke conventional medicine, but not for being too scientific, as had naturopaths before them. Rather, they complained that doctors paid too little attention to medicine's own nutritional discoveries.

Naturopathy was now on an entirely new footing. The older schools of naturopathy had closed down, but in 1978 a new one opened in Seattle: the John Bastyr College of Naturopathic Medicine (now known as Bastyr University). This school has been a strong and responsible voice for the new scientific incarnation of naturopathy.

Nonetheless, the scientific transformation of naturopathy is not yet complete. The science acceptable to naturopathic practitioners tends to be less solid than what conventional practitioners require. And while both fields resort to guesswork and speculation at times, on the naturopathic side the guesses are a bit wilder and the speculative leaps longer.

Furthermore, despite the best efforts of the more scientific of naturopaths, this field is still highly prone to fads and the influence of the bandwagon effect. Naturopaths at Bastyr University and elsewhere seem to be striving to "clean up naturopathy's act" and help it to become authentically scientific, but much work still remains to be done.

MODERN NATUROPATHY

Gone from the modern incarnation of naturopathy is the emphasis on treatment by sun, air, and water, and other aspects of the "nature cure." Presently, vitamins and other extracted food supplements are pillars of naturopathic treatment. Herbs are also important, but they have been transformed from concoctions of whole leaves and barks into standardized extracts amenable to objective testing. Their use is no longer based simply on traditional wisdom; now they are justified in terms of double-blind scientific studies.

Modern scientific naturopathy still focuses a great deal of attention on diet. However, the older principles of fasting and eating raw foods have diminished in popularity. Naturopaths continue to promote low-fat, high-fiber, semivegetarian diets such as the earliest naturopaths recommended—but by now, even the AMA recommends the same.

Not everyone is happy that naturopathic medicine is becoming so acceptably scientific. This is especially the case with those whose interest in naturopathy developed under the influence of the 1960s, a time when the original principles of naturopathy were being rediscovered and further expanded into the ecology movement.

When those new converts to the ideals of natural living looked at vitamins, they had much the same reaction as had Jethro Kloss—they recoiled. They perceived vitamins to be just another species of pills. It was not more pills they wanted, nor new scientifically approved diets, but a way of life that was in itself closer to nature.

For decades, this attitude was reflected in the structure of a new kind of store: the "natural food co-op." Unlike health food stores, these shops refused to sell vitamins, and concentrated more on the traditional principles of simple living and eating. This distinction began to break down in the late 1980s, as natural food stores bowed to public pressure and began to sell vitamins.

For good or ill, naturopathy is increasingly becoming yet another branch of the Western scientific tradition. It remains to be discovered where naturopathy will go in the future. It may become absorbed into conventional medicine, as that department dedicated to the study of food and plant-based methods of treatment. Or perhaps the tide will turn again, in yet another surge of the back-to-nature impulse.

Three major methods are used by practitioners of modern naturopathic medicine: herbal treatment, food supplement therapy, and dietary modification. The following subsections will explain these in depth, as well as warn against some common naturopathic fads.

HERBAL MEDICINE

From the very beginning, herbal treatment has been a favorite tool of naturopathically inspired practitioners. Of course, conventional medicine has also derived many of its drugs from plant sources, but there is a significant difference between an herb and a drug made from an herb. Consider the story of Kelly Freland.

On her first visit, this forty-three-year-old manager of an ecological services firm got down to business quickly: "Isn't there something natural I could take," she asked me, "instead of this drug?" She held up an asthma inhaler with distaste, as if it were a ten-day-old dead fish. "I hate putting this kind of stuff in my body," she said, making a face. "I'd much rather take an herb or something like that."

She handed me the inhaler to examine. "It's interesting that you should be taking this particular drug," I replied. "It's made from an herb. Did you know that?" She looked at me incredulously. "This asthma drug, Intal, comes from the Mediterranean herb khella," I continued. "Khella is a plant that has been used since at least the days of the pharaohs of Egypt."

I handed the inhaler back to her and she examined it with a friendlier eye. "So the white stuff in here is just ground up herb?" she asked.

"Not exactly. The inventor of Intal extracted a certain ingredient from khella, the one he thought was the most active. Unfortunately, he found that while it did help asthma, in effective doses it also caused nausea, dizziness, and other side effects. So he experimented with chemical modifications of the extract until he found a form that worked for asthma but caused no side effects."

"So I was right after all," Kelly said, a bit smugly. "Even though it originally came from an herb, it isn't natural anymore. Its been through chemical laboratories and turned into something else. Better, they call it. Why do doctors have to mess with things, thinking they can improve on nature? I'm sure the whole herb is better than the drug."

This interchange captures the difference between conventional medicine's approach to plant-based medicines, and the attitude inspired by naturopathy. Medical doctors know that herbs can be potent. In fact, pharmaceutical companies are scouring the rain forests to discover new drugs before the plants that contain them become extinct. They are also interviewing indigenous healers to get leads on promising treatments.

However, medical researchers believe that if an herb possesses medicinal powers it does so accidentally. From the point of view of evolutionary biology, plants develop chemicals that affect mammals only as a way of fending off grazing deer and other herbivores. These substances are meant to cause poisoning or at least to taste bad—not to heal. Since medical researchers believe that the medicinal powers of an herb are accidental, they always try to identify one particular active ingredient that accounts for the beneficial effect. From their point of view, it is probable that only one accidentally effective ingredient will be found in any one herb.

This attitude is totally different from the traditional herbalist's perspective on medicinal herbs. As Kloss said in *Back to Eden,* "Herbs are nature's remedies, and have been put here by an all-wise Creator." In other words, herbs were created for the express purpose of healing humans and beasts. Therefore, all the constituents of medicinal herbs are important, because they were packaged together by God. Herbalists believe that herbs should be taken as nearly whole as possible, rather than refined down to a single chemical.

Neither of these two viewpoints is right or wrong. They differ because each is based on a radically different approach to life.

Objectively speaking, it is true that some herbs seem to work better when taken whole. For example, uva-ursi (or bearberry) is a plant whose leaves are commonly used by herbalists to treat bladder infections. Studies have shown that extracts of the whole herb are more effective than the single "active ingredient" arbutin.

Scientists would attribute this difference in effectiveness to mere chance. They would say that by some accident of evolution the uva-ursi leaf possesses more than one active principle. But herbalists would nod their heads with satisfaction and say, "What else do you expect? Uva-ursi is meant to heal bladder infections, so every one of its ingredients is important. If you use whole herbs, the side effects will be less and the intended effect will be stronger."

However, the reverse is also sometimes true. The decongestant Sudafed, for example, causes less nervousness and heart palpitations than ephedra, the plant from which its main ingredient is extracted. Similarly, aspirin causes less stomach irritation than equivalent doses of white willow bark, aspirin's antecedent.

But in reality all such examples are beside the point. People who prefer herbs do not actually expect them to work better than drugs. What matters most is that herbs *feel* natural and wholesome. The driving force behind interest in herbology is aesthetic and spiritual, not coldly rational.

A Brief History of Herbology

Herbal treatment possesses an immensely old tradition. What we call conventional medicine is a newborn baby by comparison. Far back into prehistory and in every part of the world, healers have used medicinal plants to treat a great variety of afflictions.

Herbology in Europe was a traditional women's art from ancient times until the thirteenth century. The practice of healing was then taken over by graduates of male-only medical schools and members of barber-surgeon guilds. Women herbalists and midwives came to be persecuted as witches.

From that time on, most professional physicians ignored herbal treatment. Nonetheless, individuals continued to grow herbs for their own families. The naturopaths of the 1880s and early 1900s tried to revive herbology as an active practice of medicine, but the rise of powerful and effective drugs eventually suppressed interest in herbal treatment. Herbology again became popular during the 1960s, in line with the back-to-nature movement of that time. Since then, numerous books have been published on the subject, and stores specializing in the sale of herbs have proliferated.

Most often, herbs in America are sold as food supplements. Technically, it is illegal to recommend an herb as a treatment for anything—to do so is to prescribe an unapproved drug. In practice, however, herbs are widely used in this country to treat a variety of conditions, with estimated annual sales exceeding $1.3 billion.

It is interesting to note that herbology in the Western world is rather similar to conventional Western medicine in the following sense: both are disease-oriented. That is, in Western herbology a certain herb is used for a certain disease.

Oriental herbology is far different. As will be described in chapter 6, Eastern herbal approaches are far more holistic.

Modern Western herbology has divided into two branches: the use of standardized herbal extracts and the use of raw herbs. The latter is closest to the ancient tradition of herbology; the former is a far more precise and scientific method.

Standardized Extracts

Standardized herbal extracts are popular in Europe and are becoming increasingly so in the United States as well. The purpose of standardization is to overcome the problem of variability in the potency of raw herbs. The strength of a particular batch of herbs can vary with the weather, the soil in which the herbs were grown, and the variety of seed used. Therefore, it is hard to know exactly what dose to prescribe.

This difficulty can be overcome by making an extract of the whole herb and boiling off the liquid until the concentration of some ingredient reaches a certain percentage. The extract is then made into tablets or capsules, and the concentration is printed on the label. Herbalists can prescribe such herbs in terms of a total daily dose of an extract standardized to a given concentration of ingredients.

Although extracts are no longer whole herbs, they are not as refined as are chemical drugs extracted from herbs. The method of extraction used for standardized herbal products leaves most of the original ingredients intact.

A great advantage of standardized extracts is that they can be studied in double-blind controlled experiments, just like drugs. Many such studies have been performed, often involving a hundred or more participants, making them reasonably convincing in scientific terms.

Prescribing scientifically evaluated standardized herbal extracts is an accepted medical practice in Europe. The oil of the saw palmetto, for example, is widely used as a treatment for prostate enlargement in France, to the tune of $300 million annually. Studies have shown it is as effective as drugs used to treat enlarged prostates, with substantially fewer side effects. Similarly, gingko extract is popular in Germany as a proven treatment for short-term memory loss. There are many more such examples. Typically, these herbs produce few side effects compared to drugs.

European regulatory agencies are fairly liberal when it comes to approving herbs. In the United States, an herb could not be marketed as a treatment for a specific illness unless it passed the same regulatory process the FDA requires for pharmaceuticals. This typically costs more than $200 million per drug. Since herbs cannot be patented, there simply is no incentive for any company to spend that kind of money. Therefore, standardized herbal extracts are not labeled as effective for any specific conditions in the United States. They are simply sold as "supplements to the diet."

Raw Herbs

The traditional village herbalist did not use herbal extracts. She wandered over the fields to gather herbs where they grew wild. These she boiled into decoctions, made into poultices, distilled into syrups, bottled as tinctures, or dried to preserve them for future needs.

Through close observation, traditional herbalists developed many subtle distinctions. For a given problem, they preferred herbs that grew on the certain side of a mountain or were harvested at a specific date in the season. They also took note of the condition of the soil in which the herb grew, paid attention to the other plants growing around it, and considered the influence of recent weather conditions on the herb's potency.

While not as objective as actual standardization, detailed observations of this type were the practical equivalent. Traditional herbal prescription required much craft and experience.

Since the 1960s, numerous herbalists have attempted to revive this venerable form of healing. Among them is Rosemary Gladstar. She teaches classes in herbology and holds retreats and herb walks dedicated to the preparation of "wildcrafted" herbs and foods. (These are plants found in the woods, rather than grown in cultivated fields. Many herbalists consider wild herbs to be more potent than their domesticated cousins.)

Gladstar loves herbs passionately and reveres them. She cultivates an appreciation of the smell, taste, texture, and appearance of herbs, and likes to fondle them, wear them, and decorate her home with them. At one of her seminars she ate elderberry pancakes for breakfast, drank root beer brewed from Oregon grape and sassafras, and wore clothes dyed with bark and root extracts.

I remember watching her identify plants growing beside the trail. Gladstar stroked the leaves affectionately, and told reverent stories of cures in the manner one might use to recount the exploits of an admired friend.

She also provides personal herbal consultations. She pays attention to the minutest aspects of the case and prescribes herbal remedies specific to the last detail. She also makes suggestions regarding diet and exercise, and requests frequent phone consultations to follow the progress of recovery.

I have met several patients who reported marvelous cures through her work. A woman of fifty told me that Gladstar had yanked her back from the verge of a cancerous death through a vile herbal regimen more severe in its purgative effects than chemotherapy. Another told of a uterine fibroid that melted away under the influence of burdock and motherwort. A man of eighty explained that he had healed serious periodontal disease by brushing his teeth with myrrh and goldenseal. (I visited Gladstar myself for treatment of asthma, but unfortunately without any luck. This shows again that even highly competent practitioners of alternative medicine do not succeed in every case.)

In her many lectures and correspondence courses, Gladstar criticizes attempts to make herbology scientific. She fears that herbology is on its way to becoming just like conventional medicine. She would prefer her field to be sustained as a traditional art based on the loving, intuitive study of herbs. Those who agree with Rosemary Gladstar will avoid standardized herbal extracts, and instead utilize herbs in a form as close as possible to their natural state.

How Well Do Herbs Really Work?

Unfortunately, herbs do not work as well as many would like to believe. Compared to the dramatic powers of drugs, herbs are usually fairly subtle. Both their effects and their side effects are equally mild.

I first discovered this in the 1970s, while working as an organic farmer at a commune. Near the kitchen was a cabinet of medicinal herbs, frequently replenished through the gathering of wild herbs from the surrounding acreage. Like other residents of the commune, I enthusiastically embraced this fragrant form of medicine, and attempted to use it to treat my own health problems. I tried grindelia and mullein for my asthma, treated my colds with cayenne and garlic, and attempted to improve my various digestive difficulties with barberry and slippery elm. I soon started to grow and collect herbs and began to study their traditional uses.

It was a frustrating experience. Like many others who have experimented with Western herbology, I discovered that herbs used according to traditional indications seem to fail fairly frequently. There are some exceptions. Goldenseal reliably treats minor skin infections, uva-ursi can alleviate bladder infections in their very early stages, aloe vera seems to speed burn healing, and cramp bark tea relieves menstrual cramps. But in many other cases raw herbs fail to do what they're supposed to do.

Standardized herbal extracts seem to work somewhat better. Perhaps this is because the dosages used are higher than those easily obtained in dried herbs. Table 4-1 is a partial list of standardized herbal extracts that work reasonably well in real life.

Occasionally an herbal treatment proves to be more effective for a particular individual than any currently available medication. For example, I have seen a patient with uncontrollable congestive heart failure respond almost overnight to hawthorn extract. But most of the time the effects of herbs are relatively modest. Herbal treatment is usually most useful for relatively mild conditions. But because it produces so few side effects, when it works it is often distinctly preferable to drug treatment.

Are Herbs Safe?

The margin of safety of many herbs is roughly comparable to that of broccoli. Some herbs are toxic in very high doses, but safe when used as recommended. Those few that are potentially toxic even at therapeutic doses are either banned from sale or sold with warnings attached. Virtually all drugs are more dangerous than the overwhelming majority of herbs.

Table 4-1

Reasonably effective standardized herbal extracts.

Herb	Uses
Butcher's-broom	Varicose veins
Cayenne	Postherpetic neuralgia
Feverfew	Migraine headaches
Garlic	Hypertension, high cholesterol
Ginger	Nausea, motion sickness
Gingko	Short-term memory loss, peripheral and cerebral vascular insufficiency
Gotu kola	Varicose veins
Gugulu	High cholesterol
Gymnema sylvestre	Adult-onset diabetes
Hawthorne	Hypertension, angina, minor arrythmias
Kava	Insomnia, anxiety
Licorice	Peptic ulcers, herpes, eczema
Milk thistle	Hepatitis, gallstones
Peppermint	Irritable bowel syndrome
St. John's-wort	Depression, insomnia
Saw palmetto	Benign prostatic hypertrophy
Turmeric	Anti-inflammatory
Uva-ursi	Urinary tract infections

How to Obtain Advice on Herbology

Herbology is practiced by naturopaths, chiropractors, nutritionists, herbologists, alternative M.D.s, and, informally, by employees of health food stores. Although there is no single standard for the certification of herbalists, several organizations of practitioners exist. Some are listed in the Resources section.

Many books are available on the subject of herbs. Some of the best are listed in the Resources section.

VITAMINS AND OTHER FOOD SUPPLEMENTS

The use of vitamins and food supplements is another major branch of naturopathy, and probably the most widely available and well-known of all alternative treatments. Practically every issue of every popular magazine contains recommendations such as antioxidants for preventing cancer, vitamin E to treat fibrocystic breast disease, and "flushless" niacin for lowering cholesterol.

There is no longer any doubt that food supplements can be effective. The textbook *Nutritional Influences on Illness,* by Melvyn Werbach, M.D., includes over six hundred pages of research references regarding the use of these substances. While some of these studies were tiny, poorly performed, or otherwise inadequate, many were reasonably large and carried out under the supervision of medical researchers at prestigious universities.

This is an impressive collection of studies, especially given the fact that it is very difficult to raise money to study food supplements. Like herbs, they usually cannot be patented. Drug companies are the main source of funds for such research, and, naturally, they would rather pay to study substances on which they stand to make a profit.

Nonetheless, enough good research exists to prove that materials derived from foods can be effective in the treatment of various diseases. From niacin for high cholesterol to glucosamine sulfate for arthritis pain, numerous food supplements have been shown useful in the treatment of diseases. Many produce significantly fewer side effects than drugs of comparable effectiveness.

In the old days, medical doctors resisted the notion of vitamin therapy, partly because alternative practitioners were pushing it so hard. But those times have changed. Conventional medicine now readily embraces vitamins and supplements of proven efficacy. Established conventional medical journals now commonly refer to the use of vitamins in treatment, calling them "medications," and listing them as options along with prescription and nonprescription drugs.

Being less conservative by nature, alternative practitioners do not feel they must wait for full scientific proof before recommending food supplements. Even a shred of evidence may be enough for them to try it. Sometimes these speculative uses of supplements are later validated by solid research. Often, however, the supplements prescribed widely one year disappear the next, when contrary evidence appears. (The same happens with drugs, but not quite so frequently.)

The Two Uses of Food Supplements

Food supplements can be used in two ways: at relatively low doses to make up for an inadequate diet ("nutritional medicine"), or in immense doses to produce a specific therapeutic effect ("megadose therapy").

Nutritional Medicine. Studies have shown that deficiencies of many essential nutrients are surprisingly common among Americans. Some of the most frequently cited deficiencies include calcium, folic acid, iron, magnesium, zinc, and vitamins A, B6, C, and E. Senior citizens often suffer from additional deficiencies.

Even conventional medicine agrees that those who do not eat a balanced diet can benefit from supplementation with vitamins and minerals. But many naturopathically inclined practitioners further believe that even if dietary intake is adequate, individuals can easily develop nutritional deficits due to poor digestive absorption. They also point out that the stresses of modern life and the effects of toxic substances in the environment may cause nutritional needs to increase beyond what can easily be supplied by food. Finally, they maintain that plants grown under modern artificial conditions simply do not supply enough nutrients.

For all these reasons, many naturopaths claim that vitamin and mineral supplementation may be important for everyone, regardless of diet. Whether this is true remains a matter of controversy.

Megadose Therapy. The second and more dramatic use of food supplements employs doses far beyond any reasonable nutritional requirement. Linus Pauling's famous vitamin C recommendations are a good example of this "supranutritional" approach. The official RDA (recommended daily allowance) for vitamin C is 60 mg (milligrams) daily. Multiplying this by ten to allow for the effects of stress, imperfect absorption, and a possible antivitamin bias by the FDA, we arrive at a figure of 600 mg a day. Such a dose should be far more than enough to provide for basic dietary needs.

But Pauling and many other practitioners of vitamin therapy recommend daily doses of 4,000 to 10,000 mg. This is the equivalent of forty to a hundred oranges per day, hardly a likely nutritional need!

There are many other such examples. Modern advocates of antioxidant therapy recommend similarly high doses of vitamin C, along with heroic amounts of vitamin E and carotene. Other alternative practitioners recommend vitamin B12 at about fifteen times the recommended daily allowance to treat asthma, allergies, and fatigue. Ten times the ordinary intake of zinc is supposed to be helpful for prostate enlargement.

A related treatment method involves the use of substances present in food but not actually necessary for good nutrition. The "nonessential" amino acid gamma-aminobutyric acid (GABA) is a good example. Although the body does not require it in the diet, fairly high doses of GABA can sometimes alleviate the symptoms of anxiety.

How Well Do Supplements Actually Work?

In cases of actual nutritional deficiency, basic vitamin and mineral supplementation can improve overall health and prevent disease. But only occasionally does purely nutritional supplementation help specific health problems.

Megadose supplement therapy, however, can be highly effective for identified medical conditions. I've seen many remarkable results, ranging from dramatic treatment of chronic anxiety with GABA through successful reduction of blood pressure through the use of coenzyme Q10. Perhaps the most impressive result was a patient crippled by osteoarthritis and doubled over in pain from the stomach ulcers her arthritis medication had raised. After two months of taking glucosamine sulfate, she was pain free and playing tennis. Table 4-2 summarizes some of the most clinically effective of the megadose supplement methods.

Despite their respectable effectiveness, megadose supplements are usually not as powerful as drugs. Supplement therapy alone is seldom adequate for conditions of a severe nature. However, even when drugs are required, food supplements may be useful as adjuncts to therapy and may sometimes reduce the

Table 4-2

Reasonably effective megadose supplements.

Supplement	Uses
Coenzyme Q10	Hypertension
GABA	Anxiety
Gamma-oryzanol	Menopause symptoms
Glucosamine sulfate	Osteoarthritis
L-lysine	Cold sores
"Nonflush" niacin	High cholesterol
Vitamin B6	Premenstrual syndrome
Vitamin B12	Asthma, fatigue
Vitamin C	Cold symptoms
Vitamin E	Fibrocystic breast disease, menopause symptoms
Zinc	Prostate enlargement, prostatitis, chronic boils

amount of medication required. For example, patients with severe hypertension can often reduce doses of side-effect-ridden drugs by adding side-effect-free supplements to their regime. Patients with moderate hypertension can often do away with drugs entirely.

These comments apply to the best of the supplement methods. Unfortunately, the marketplace is flooded with exaggerated claims. Food supplement medicine is an extremely faddish field, and one that is packed with hype. In my experience, considerably less than one in twenty of the supplements advertised really do anything.

Health food stores and supplement manufacturers are commercial enterprises. For them, scientific studies are marketing tools, not keys to discovering the truth. A close look will often reveal that much of what passes for research really doesn't amount to much.

For example, consider the substances known as antioxidants. According to innumerable magazine articles—indeed, entire books—vitamins E, A, and C prevent cancer and retard aging. Many people have come to believe this as an established fact. But the theory that links these substances to their supposed benefits is actually an extended chain of maybes. It goes as follows:

Epidemiological studies have shown that people who eat more fruits and vegetables live longer and have a lower incidence of cancer than those who do not (fact). In particular, foods in the broccoli family seem to have an anticancer effect (fact). Fruits and vegetables contain relatively high levels of vitamins E, A, and C (fact). Maybe these are the active ingredients in fruits and vegetables (an unproved supposition. What about the ten thousand other interesting substances in these foods?).

On a molecular level, vitamins E, A, and C neutralize other molecules called oxidants (fact). These oxidants may be involved in aging and the origin of cancer (hypothesis). These vitamins' molecular properties may mean that they are important players in a high-stakes fight the body may be waging against these oxidants (hypothesis). Supplementing these vitamins to very high levels may help win this fight. (This is the "more is better" theory.)

From this chain of maybes, some conclude that antioxidants may be the health-promoting ingredients in fruits and vegetables, and that by taking immense quantities of them, a person may live longer.

That's a truckload of maybes! This argument is really no more than a possible starting point for further investigation. To research the antioxidant hypothesis properly, experimenters would have to dose a large group of subjects with these vitamins and follow them for many years, and at the same time follow an equally large group identical in every way except for the vitamin treatment.

No such study has ever shown that antioxidants prevent cancer. There even seems to be some evidence that vitamin A (as synthetic carotene) can increase cancer risk in certain cases. The cancer-preventing effects of fruits and vegetables may be due to something completely different, not the vitamins they contain.

In the absence of confirming studies, the antioxidant hypothesis is mere speculation. Consuming these vitamins probably won't hurt. It might make sense as a just-in-case measure.

By the same token, evidence does exist proving the benefits of supplements. I recommend maintaining a high index of skepticism toward all new supplements on the market, and toward new uses of old products. Most of these will prove to be will-o'-the-wisps. But if a supplement is still popular five years after it was introduced, it may be worth looking into. Time tends to clear away nonsense.

How to Obtain Supplement Recommendations

Because of the haze of faddism and commercialism, it can be difficult to discern the most truly useful food supplements. I suggest obtaining recommendations from a practitioner who has had wide experience in their use and actually pays attention to the results. Unfortunately, there are relatively few of these.

Virtually every kind of alternative practitioner recommends supplements. In my experience only a minority of those who prescribe supplements maintain an attitude of careful pragmatism. Too many jump on the bandwagon of fads and make recommendations based on pure speculation. Responsible practitioners should pay attention to whether their methods actually work and quit using those approaches that come up short. The sad fact is that many prescribers of supplements seem not to learn from feedback. They continue to recommend clinically ineffective supplements, and remain blissfully unaware of doing so.

Of course there are responsible supplement prescribers too. Some of the best are graduates of naturopathic schools, such as Bastyr University in Seattle.

In the Resources section at the end of this book, I note several books that contain clinically grounded advice on the use of supplements. Also, in section V I recommend supplements that are actually useful for treating a number of conditions.

Dangers of Supplements

Although incidences of permanent injury through supplement treatment are rare, some supplements can be toxic when taken in excessive doses. Table 4-3 lists some of the most important risks to consider. Melvyn Werbach's *Nutritional Influences on Illness* contains a comprehensive listing of the known side effects of food supplements.

Table 4-3

Risks of supplementation.

Supplement	Possible Side Effects
Copper	Confusion, fatigue, depression
Folic acid	Seizures
Germanium	Kidney injury
L-lysine	Increased cholesterol
Manganese	Neurological disorders, hypertension
Niacin	Liver injury
PABA (para-aminobenzoic acid)	Impaired liver function
Phenylalanine	Hypertension
Vitamin A	Liver injury, bone changes, many other symptoms
Vitamin B6	Peripheral neuropathy
Vitamin C	Diarrhea, kidney stones
Vitamin D	Hypercalcemia with kidney damage and calcium deposits in various tissues
Zinc	Impaired immune function

Besides these side effects, there is a real problem with quality control in the retail supplement world. I have read many disturbing surveys that show widespread discrepancies between what it says on a food supplement label and the actual contents. The only way to verify the potency of a given supplement is to read an independent laboratory analysis. The better supplement manufacturers will make this information available on request. In the future, I hope that the supplement industry will take the enlightened step of adopting voluntary quality control standards. Failing that, the FDA may need to get involved.

Is This Really Alternative Medicine?

While food supplements can definitely treat diseases and promote good health, they fulfill few of the ideals of alternative medicine. This objection is especially strong in the case of megadose supplements, but it applies to nutritional supplementation as well.

One objection is that vitamins aren't natural. They are refined, processed products. When a chemical such as digitalis is extracted from the plant foxglove it is called a drug, not an herb. Similarly, when vitamin C is extracted from rose hips, it should no longer be thought of as a food. It is now a chemical produced from a food source. White sugar is extracted from a natural food too, but it is not usually considered a natural nutritional supplement.

Rose hips are a food. Crystalline vitamin C from rose hips or any other source is still crystalline vitamin C. The expression "a natural vitamin" means about as much as "natural white sugar."

Further objections apply to megadose treatment. Just like drugs, megadose supplements must be taken on an ongoing basis to produce their effect. They cannot truly "get to the root of the problem and heal from within." Also, to take supplements in doses that go radically beyond nutritional needs is to violate the ideal of keeping close to nature.

Additional evidence of the nonalternative nature of supplement therapy may be found in the fact that conventional medicine itself is quite comfortable (in principle) with the method. The nutritional use of vitamins and minerals was pioneered by medical researchers, not naturopaths. And numerous high-dose supplement methods are being investigated at major medical centers. They will be incorporated into standard practice as fast as they are solidly proved effective. Large doses of niacin, for example, are already widely prescribed by physicians to lower cholesterol.

For all these reasons, those who wish truly alternative treatment should probably look elsewhere than to megavitamin therapy.

DIET

Methods of treatment involving changes in diet have always been a central theme of naturopathy. Early naturopaths believed that fruits, vegetables, and whole grains were what humans ate "in the natural state," and that such foods were imbued with natural vitality and life energy. Any adulteration or refinement of these foods was seen as reducing their aliveness and diminishing their health-giving properties. As Jethro Kloss said, "When fruits, grains, nuts and vegetables are eaten in their natural state and not perverted and robbed of their life-giving properties in their preparation, health, beauty, and happiness will be the sure reward." The original naturopaths also believed that meat was essentially toxic, a kind of dead food that inevitably caused illness.

In contrast, conventional medicine has historically paid relatively little attention to diet. Medical doctors pooh-poohed naturopathic dietary recommendations for decades and proclaimed that what a person ate usually didn't matter much. Only in the 1980s did the medical establishment begin to take seriously the notion that diet is a primary influence on health. By now, of course, the results of large-scale epidemiological studies have shown that diet, along with exercise, is of central importance in preventing nearly all the major health problems of twentieth-century America: such conditions as breast cancer, colon cancer, prostate cancer, heart disease, and strokes. No other medical intervention can do as much to maintain a state of good health.

By a strange chance, the diet that old-time naturopaths proposed on philosophical grounds has turned out to match exactly the low-fat, high-fiber diet high in fresh fruits and vegetables that medical science now recommends. Somehow those naturopaths managed to discover the fundamental laws of healthy diet. That they did so without the benefit of research demonstrates that science is not the only possible source of knowledge. Nonetheless, it is nice that science has finally confirmed what naturopaths felt intuitively.

Although medical doctors now recognize that diet is important, it still goes against the grain of their thinking to dwell on the subject. Doctors customarily delegate dietary issues to dietitians, preferring to spend their time on more interesting topics, like the latest drug. Even those doctors who do feel inclined to recommend dietary changes often get burned out and give up. The problem is that too many patients fail to change their eating habits. Dietary change is difficult and arduous, and the habits of a lifetime are not easily altered. After doctors have lectured a couple of hundred patients on the benefits of good diet, and only a handful have made any changes, the doctors may begin to consider the effort a waste of breath.

Alternative practitioners ordinarily spend considerable time counseling changes in diet. They have a considerable advantage, however, in that patients who seek out alternative treatment are more commonly willing to make difficult lifestyle modifications.

Past the Medically Approved Diet

Alternative practitioners generally go further in their recommendations than what scientific medicine has come to accept. In addition to meat and fat, they condemn food preservatives and the artificial fertilizers, pesticides, antibiotics, and hormones involved in modern farming. Foods raised without these influences are called "organically grown," and are favored by all proponents of alternative medicine. These preferences show the obvious influence of the back-to-nature movement.

Natural food adherents argue that chemicals are dangerous unless proved safe. In contrast, medical doctors instinctively trust chemicals and tend to assume that additives are safe until proved otherwise. These opposing viewpoints are based on fundamental philosophical differences described earlier. There is no point arguing about it one way or the other; the desire for organically grown food is an intuitive principle more than a rational one. But maybe the naturopathic intuition will once more prove right.

Beyond Organic Foods

Alternative dietary recommendations often go even further than organically raised meat and produce. From this point on, the various popular food theories become remarkably contradictory.

A highly influential naturopathic concept dating back a century or more claims that raw fruits and vegetables contain more life force, not to mention vitamins, enzymes, and proteins than do cooked foods. As recently as 1994, a proponent of this "raw food theory" announced that "the greatest enemy of man is the cooking stove!"

Another popular theory, macrobiotics, bans raw foods as unhealthy and considers them a cause of illnesses such as multiple sclerosis and rheumatoid arthritis. This theory insists that all vegetables should be cooked.

Other discrepancies abound. The following dietary rules may be found in one or another food theory: Spicy food is bad. Cayenne pepper promotes health. Eating nothing but oranges is healthy. Citrus fruits are too acidic. Fruits are the ideal food. Fruit causes *Candida* infections. Milk is good only for young cows. Pasteurized milk is even worse. Boiled milk "is the food of the gods." Fermented foods, such as sauerkraut, are essentially rotten. Fermented foods aid digestion. Sweets are bad. Honey is nature's most perfect food. Vinegar is a poison. Apple cider vinegar cures most illnesses. Proteins should not be combined with starches. Aduki beans and brown rice should always be cooked together.

The list could be continued for many pages. I once planned to write a universal cookbook for eating theorists. Each food would come complete with a citation from one system or authority claiming it the most divine edible ever created, and another, from an opposing view, damning it as the worst pestilence one human being ever fed to another. Medical doctors are often maligned for failing to study dietary theory. But, which theory should they study?

Personally, I have had considerable exposure to the intensity of food theories. When I became a cook at a large commune in the late 1970s, I discovered that I had unknowingly waded into a vast sea of dietary beliefs. All communes tend to attract idealists; this one attracted food idealists. I was required to cook several separate meals at once to satisfy the insistent and conflicting demands of our members.

The main entree was always vegetarian, but a small but vocal group insisted on an optional serving of meat. Since many vegetarians would not eat from pots and pans "contaminated by flesh," this meat had to be cooked in a separate kitchen. The cooks also had to satisfy the lacto-ovo-vegetarians, or vegans, who eschewed all milk and egg products. The rights of the no-garlic, no-onion Hindu-influenced crowd could not be neglected either. They believed onion-family foods provoked sexual desire.

For the raw "foodniks" (and young children), we always laid out trays of sliced raw vegetables. Once, a visitor tried to convince me that chopping a vegetable would destroy its "etheric field," but I chased him out of the kitchen with a huge Chinese cleaver. The macrobiotic adherents clamored for cooked vegetables—free from "deadly nightshade" plants such as tomatoes, potatoes, bell peppers, and eggplants. Some of our members insisted on eating only fruits and vegetables in season, while others intemperately demanded oranges in January.

Besides so many variations on the food we served, many opinions clashed on the manner in which it should be prepared. Nothing could be boiled in aluminum, ever. Most everyone agreed to that—except the gourmet cooks, who said that only aluminum would spread the heat satisfactorily.

By consensus, we always steamed vegetables in a minimal amount of water, to avoid throwing away precious vitamins. Certain enthusiasts would hover around the kitchen and volunteer to drink the darkish liquids left behind. About washing vegetables, controversy swirled. Some firmly believed that vital substances clung just under the skins of most vegetables, which would be lost in washing. Others felt that a host of evil pollutants adhered to the same surfaces, and needed to be vigorously scrubbed away. One visitor said that she always dipped her vegetables in bleach. She gave such a convincing argument that we might have adopted the principle at once were it not for a fortuitous bleach shortage.

Although at the time the inconsistency of what I encountered bothered me very much, in retrospect I find all these experiences amusing. I now recognize that, like all aspects of alternative medicine, food medicine is prone to extremes.

What Approach to Diet Is the Best?

There is no problem finding practitioners (and neighbors) willing to make dietary recommendations. The difficult question is deciding which school to follow.

Innumerable books have been written on proper diet. Since they all disagree with one another on specifics, however, a trip to a bookstore will more likely be a source of confusion than enlightenment.

The bulletin boards of natural food or health food stores list macrobiotic counselors, lacto-ovo-vegetarian cooking teachers, certified nutritional advisors, and usually a few chiropractors, massage therapists, and "energy" healers. But again, since they all disagree on everything but the low-fat, semivegetarian diet that everyone endorses, individual choice is still necessary.

I wish I could say that some of these dietary beliefs were true and others were wrong. Unfortunately, reality is not so black-and-white. Different approaches work for different people. Which path to take, if any, will probably ultimately come down to personal intuition and trial and error.

Can Dietary Changes Cure Illness?

Despite all the contradictions, specific methods of dietary manipulation can be highly effective. Almost every week I meet a patient who has successfully cured himself of one disease or another through dietary manipulation. I've seen numerous children whose frequent ear infections were easily cured by simply removing milk from their diets. Many cases of chronic fatigue, low resistance to illness, mental confusion, arthritis, allergies, asthma, and digestive disorders also seem to respond readily to dietary manipulation. Even such terrible problems as multiple sclerosis, lupus, and cancer occasionally go into remission through food therapy.

The dietary changes used to promote these recoveries have ranged widely, from antiallergy and anti-yeast approaches through raw food, the Gerson diet, and macrobiotics. Among the most peculiar regimes I have ever encountered are the Jonathan apple fast and the steak-and-orange diet.

Like every method of healing, the effectiveness of dietary change is variable. I have definitely seen more failures than successes, and sometimes changing the diet can make a person get sicker.

Because the number of possible specific approaches to diet is so large, it is not possible to undertake a survey of them all. But I would like to go into some depth regarding one of the most effective specific dietary methods, as well as point out a danger inherent in every therapeutic approach to eating: the possibility that it can become an obsession.

The Food Allergy Diet

The concept of food allergies did not exist in traditional naturopathy, but it has become a popular concern among those who practice naturopathic methods today. Diets based on avoiding allergenic or "trigger" foods are widely recommended for many conditions, from chronic fatigue and frequent infections to obesity and arthritis.

The concept of food allergy per se is accepted by conventional medicine, but medical doctors are usually only concerned with dramatic and obvious allergic reactions, such as the nearly instantaneous breakout into hives that can occur with shellfish allergies. More subtle reactions usually do not interest conventional practitioners, following the general rule that conventional medicine does not like to deal with vague, indefinable complaints.

Naturopathic practitioners, however, are not deterred by vagueness. They take a great interest in identifying foods that cause elusive and subjective symptoms. The branch of naturopathy concerned with food allergies is often called clinical ecology. According to Joseph Pizzorno and Michael Murray's *Textbook of Natural Medicine,* the book used to train naturopaths at Bastyr University, advocates of this approach claim that food allergies are the leading cause of most undiagnosed symptoms.

Actually, *food sensitivity* is a more accurate choice of words than *food allergy.* Some foods cause problems even though a true allergic response to them is impossible. Sugar is a good example. It is impossible to be allergic to sugar, because the bloodstream is always full of sugar. But some patients develop numerous symptoms when they eat sugary foods. Thus, they are sensitive to sugar, although not literally allergic.

Naturopaths use a variety of methods for determining food allergies. Many laboratory tests are available, but their reliability is a matter of controversy. The only method on which all naturopathic practitioners agree consists of an elimination diet followed by food challenges.

A patient using this technique begins by going on a highly restricted diet, usually consisting of only a few foods known to seldom cause allergies. Turkey, white rice, and sweet potatoes are popular. After a few weeks a number of chronic symptoms should begin to clear. (If they don't, it either means that food allergies were not the problem in the first place, or that the patient is sensitive to one of the permitted foods.)

Once optimum clearing is achieved, various foods are added back to the diet, one at a time. The patient keeps a journal, paying particular attention to reactions such as increased pulse rate, sneezing, headache, increased fatigue, or a return of the original symptoms. This process eventually results in the identification of all problem foods. Patients can subsequently avoid these foods and thereby hope to improve their health.

The food allergy method sometimes works splendidly. I have seen numerous people use it to recover from a wide variety of problems, including chronic fatigue, depression, frequent infections, digestive problems, joint pain, asthma, eczema, obesity, migraine headaches, and even serious diseases such as rheumatoid arthritis or multiple sclerosis.

However, not everyone so benefits. Many people show no particular improvement after months of effort. Furthermore, even when it works, trigger-food avoidance exacts a substantial cost for its results. This method can cause social isolation by putting most ordinary menus off-limits. Also, through the immense attention they must pay to small matters of diet, many who work with food allergies become obsessed over what they eat. This obsession may become so pronounced that it develops into what amounts to an eating disorder.

It can be quite helpful to identify and avoid a few problematic foods. But I recommend absolute avoidance of "trigger" foods only as a last resort. An enthusiastic embrace of the method often leads to a way of life that produces more misery than the original illness.

"Orthorexia Nervosa"—
The Third Eating Disorder

Eating can become an obsession for the health-minded, no matter what their theory. I have coined the term *orthorexia nervosa* to denote this fixation on eating healthy food—*ortho,* meaning straight, correct, true; the rest of the term analogous to anorexia nervosa.

Orthorexia begins innocently, as a desire to overcome some chronic illness or to improve general health. Over time, what one eats, how much, and the consequences of dietary indiscretion come to occupy a greater and greater proportion of the day. It requires much willpower to adopt a diet that differs radically from the food habits of one's childhood and the surrounding culture. Few accomplish the change gracefully. Most must use an iron self-discipline to avoid temptation, bolstered by a hefty sense of superiority over those who eat junk food.

Soon, the act of eating pure food begins to carry pseudospiritual connotations. It comes to seem as if abstaining from refined foods was akin to dedicating one's life to serve the poor. To orthorexics, a day filled with sprouts, umeboshi plums, and amaranth biscuits feels like an interlude of heaven on earth. They feel good, noble, and righteous.

In contrast, when they slip up (which, depending on the particular theory involved, may involve anything from devouring a single peanut to consuming a gallon of Häagen-Dazs ice cream and a large pizza), they experience a fall from grace. They take upon themselves acts of penitence to remedy their giving in to carnal desire. These usually involve ever-stricter diets and fasts.

As this "kitchen spirituality" progresses, all other meaning gradually pales before food. Orthorexics will be plunged into gloom by eating a hot dog, even if their team has just won the World Series. In contrast, sadness and failure may be redeemed by extra efforts at dietary purity.

Orthorexia may reach a point where sufferers spend most of the day planning, purchasing, and eating meals. The larger part of their inner lives may be filled with resisting temptation, praising themselves for success at complying with this self-chosen regime, condemning themselves for lapses, and feeling superior to others less pure in their dietary habits.

It is this transference of all life's value into the act of eating that makes orthorexia a true eating disorder. Like anorexics and bulimics, orthorexics have projected their soul onto food. Their obsession over healthy food relieves orthorexics from seeking real meaning in their lives.

The many schools of eating, and the practitioners who promote them, seem entirely unaware that the search for healthy food can become a disorder. Indeed, natural medicine appears to actively promote orthorexia. No doubt, this is a compensation for the stance of modern medicine, which has too long largely ignored diet. However, healthy eating all too often becomes a disease in its own right, far worse than the health problems that began the cycle of fixation.

Personally, I almost never recommend radical diets, except occasionally in cases of illness so severe that it is worth restricting one's life in hopes of a cure. I concur with limiting milk, meat, sugar, and chemicals. I agree that vegetables should be eaten in large portions, along with whole grains and legumes and a minimum of meat. But, for me, to go beyond that is to go too far. Surgery may even be preferable to an extreme diet! Life is so short—it is a shame to waste time obsessing over eating.

FADS

Naturopathy is perpetually prone to the influence of fads. I'm not sure why this should be, but it is an ever present reality. Naturopathic fads consist primarily of two types: theories that explain a wide variety of illnesses, and magic substances that are supposed to cure a wide variety of illnesses. These methods persist in popularity, not because they work very well, but because they are so simple.

Candida

An example of the first kind of simple solution is the famous diagnosis known simply as *Candida,* or more formally as "the yeast syndrome." *Candida albicans* has long been known as the cause of vaginal yeast infections and infant thrush. Following the publication of Dr. William Crook's very popular book *The Yeast*

Connection, however, alternative practitioners expanded their view of what *Candida* could do.

According to Dr. Crook's theory, an excess of the common yeast *Candida* causes a wide variety of common symptoms, including fatigue, depression, sinus allergies, and frequent colds. Alternative practitioners flocked to accept this concept with great enthusiasm, probably because it involved a special diet. At the moment I write this book, it is almost impossible to complain of fatigue to a chiropractor, naturopath, alternative M.D., or nutritionist without being told, "You must have *Candida.*"

To hear many alternative practitioners talk about it, chronic *Candida* is one of the most widespread and significant health problems in the world. There is no doubt that for some people anti-yeast treatment can be quite helpful. In my experience, however, most people who use the *Candida* method obtain no improvement for their efforts. *Candida* is vastly overhyped.

I am sure that within twenty years only a small percentage of patients will be diagnosed with *Candida.* By then, something new will have taken its place, just as *Candida* replaced the formerly popular universal "cause" of fatigue: hypoglycemia.

There are many other fad theories. One of the most popular asserts that hypothyroidism that does not show up on lab tests is the cause of most illnesses; another is that intestinal parasites are the true cause of cancer. No doubt, each fad theory has a kernel of truth, but not enough to support the mountain of enthusiasm that is built on top of it.

Magic Substances

The other prevalent form of fad in naturopathy involves materials rather than theories. I call this phenomenon "magic substance worship." Because I have succumbed to it myself, I have a definite sympathy for the impulse. However, this is perhaps the most shallow form of alternative medicine. There is no depth, no art, no holism, no real understanding of healing in substance worship.

Drugs are not very romantic—I have never met a patient who idealized and extolled the virtues of, say, ibuprofen. But, in the world of alternative medicine, many people develop an almost mystical passion for bee propolis, vitamin C, or spirulina.

Since the beginning of my professional involvement with alternative medicine, probably not one month has gone by without some new marvelous material reaching my ears or my desk. These include DHEA, pycnogenol, super blue-green algae (the successor to spirulina), purple lapacho, Essiac, coenzyme Q10, colloidal silver, royal jelly, eleuthero ginseng, the Manchurian mushroom, tea-tree oil, bovine colostrum, astragalus, lobelia, superconcentrated hydrogen peroxide, and many other products.

Entire books have been written about each of these. Adherents will practically grab strangers at the airport to evangelize on behalf of their chosen material. Some substances come with speculative explanations attached. Others must be taken on faith, and are usually associated with the ancient wisdom of some distant ethnic group, such as the Aztecs, Hunzas, Tibetans, or Chinese.

The earliest magic substance I can recall is chlorophyll. Touted as a cure-all almost from the instant of its discovery, this essential plant chemical was extremely popular for a brief time. I remember a certain gum packed with chlorophyll that was sold at the counter of health food stores. It was supposed to cure headaches, allergies, ulcers, and colds. Who praises chlorophyll today (besides plants)?

Most of these healing materials possess both pedigree and personality. Lobelia, first appreciated by the Thomsonians in the last century, and rating fully twenty-eight consecutive pages in Jethro Kloss's *Back to Eden,* carries rigorous overtones of cures preceded by intense vomiting. It hearkens back to the days when "men were real men," and "taking your medicine" meant much the same, whether it was a beating or a foul herbal brew.

Colloidal silver pills, on the other hand, bear resonances of Indian purity and elegance. Long used in Ayurvedic medicine (the traditional medical system of India), silver carries a Brahminical resonance of purity and cleanliness. By swallowing what is precious, even guts can be purified! The appeal of silver is doubtless based as much on this Eastern symbolism as on silver's modern use to stop bacterial overgrowth in water purification systems.

Certain personalities are attracted to certain cures. The bitter brilliance of wheatgrass juice attracted hippies such as myself, who were rediscovering asceticism over bowls of brown rice. DHEA and DMSO (dimethylsulfoxide) appeal to the more technologically minded. Ginseng, especially in its whole form, preserved in honey, captures the imagination of those who bear a fascination for the East. If only healing were really this easy!

Two things about this habit of substance worship give me pain. First, it is so dreadfully materialistic. I do not believe that a substance is a worthy icon. When people curl themselves around a particular mystic material, they shrink their lives to the dimensions of a green liquid, a brown powder, or a food. Healing is not, and cannot be, so simple.

Second, despite my sense of what is right and good, these reverenced materials occasionally do cure! I find this appalling. According to my instinctive leanings, a medicine should work frequently or not at all. It should prove reliable or an absolute fraud. That a supplement can work rare miracles offends my sensibilities. Yet, I am often offended in just this way.

In my experience, every remedy, without exception, occasionally succeeds brilliantly. I did not realize this twenty years ago when I began to study alternative medicine. I used to believe that if one person rid himself of rheumatoid arthritis with, say, propolis, the same method should work for nearly everyone who repeats the experiment. Certainly, there might be an occasional failure. But if a substance can cure, really cure, dramatically—even once—it must be powerful medicine!

But as my experience grew, I discovered that my initial impression was incorrect. Supplements and herbs that work marvelously for one individual commonly fail miserably for a hundred others. Dramatic testimonials say nothing about rates of success.

I remember a patient named Pearl O'Shaughnessy who developed severe chronic fatigue syndrome (CFS). She had once been an athlete, but after a year of CFS she looked like she had been bedridden for years. I tried everything I knew to help her, from acupuncture and Chinese herbs to nutrition, detoxification, body-oriented psychotherapy, Rolfing, and food allergy testing. But despite my best efforts and the efforts of the sophisticated alternative practitioners to whom I sent her, after a year she was still too sick to walk more than half a block.

Then she met Dr. L. I have known Dr. L. for many years and regard him with little respect. To me, he typifies all that is wrong with alternative medicine. He jumps on every new product bandwagon and adopts all the half-baked alternative theories he comes across, failing in the least to discriminate between the solid and the ridiculous.

When Pearl came to him, Dr. L. prescribed his favorite magic substance of the season: coenzyme Q10. (That year, he was prescribing it to everyone.) It was a foolish recommendation, and I told Pearl so. Within a month of starting Dr. L.'s treatment, however, she was running ten miles a day.

Coenzyme Q10 is a substance found naturally in the mitochondria, the energy-producing centers of the cells. Dr. L. claimed that since the mitochondria help produce bodily energy, and since CoQ10 is an essential part of the mitochondria, it follows that supplementing the diet with CoQ10 will increase energy.

This is a very weak chain of reasoning. One might as well argue that since spark plugs help produce energy inside the motors of cars, ground up spark plugs should be added to the gas tanks of sluggish vehicles. The logic is absurd. It is classic pretend-science.

For Pearl, however, a week's worth of CoQ10 had sufficed to accomplish what all my sophisticated efforts could not. I couldn't argue with the results. Indeed, I was so impressed that I tried CoQ10 on all my other chronic fatigue sufferers.

It failed miserably every time. But, after seeing what it had done for Pearl, I refused to give up. Four years and dozens of patients later, I saw CoQ10 work another miracle.

Results such as this make impressive testimonials. However, they are ultimately unsatisfying. What use is a substance that only cures occasionally? Should I simply recommend that my patients start at one end of the health food store and work their way to the other?

I generally advise my patients to ignore all magic healing substances and their claims. Naturopathy and the other fields of alternative medicine have much better offerings. But healing is mysterious, and even the least sophisticated of methods will occasionally surpass the highest forms of healing.

CHAPTER 5

Homeopathy

It is with considerable hesitation that I place homeopathy in the category of scientific approaches to healing. While homeopathy's general approach is science-like, most scientists regard the field as obvious nonsense.

Unlike herbs and food supplements, homeopathic remedies contain no measurable material constituents (other than sugar). For this reason, scientists find it difficult to imagine that homeopathics can actually do anything. There seems to be some objective evidence, however, that homeopathy works. Either this evidence is wrong, or homeopathy works by means of a hitherto undiscovered force of nature.

Homeopathy was the invention of a German physician named Samuel Hahnemann (1755–1843). Disgusted with the barbaric medical practices of his day, Dr. Hahnemann sought to formulate a system of medicine much gentler than what he saw practiced around him. His method rapidly grew in popularity and spread to many countries, embraced in large part because it was so much kinder than conventional treatment.

Actually, almost any approach to medicine would have been kinder than the prevailing medical practices of Hahnemann's day. Conventional medicine at the time employed methods then described as "heroic," involving exuberant bleeding of patients, blistering of the skin, induction of vomiting with poisonous salts of antimony, and intestinal purging through mercury poisoning. It is well documented that George Washington was killed by such procedures at the hands of doctors "treating" his sore throat.

Compared to the ferocious irrationality of the medicine practiced around him, Hahnemann's approach was elegant and refined. He based homeopathy on three principles of his own invention. The first is "The Law of Similars," or "like cures like." Hahnemann felt that a substance that causes certain symptoms in a healthy individual can cure a diseased person suffering from those same symptoms if it is taken in small doses.

The second principle is "The Law of Infinitesimals." It states that the more dilute the dose of a remedy, the more powerful its effects. Third, "The Law of Chronic Disease" states that treatments like herbs or drugs (which Hahnemann called "allopathic") drive conditions deeper into the body, while homeopathic remedies based on the first two laws release these buried problems and produce true healing from within.

HOW IS HOMEOPATHY PRACTICED?

Hahnemann and his associates undertook to apply the Law of Similars by taking high doses of various substances. The results of these risky experiments (known as "provings") were carefully noted and recorded into a materia medica of possible treatments.

Hahnemann's original materia medica is still the basis of treatment today, although it has been greatly expanded. When presented with a patient, so-called "classical" or "constitutional" homeopaths take a full inventory of the patient's symptoms and personality characteristics. They then look in the materia medica to find a substance that produces similar effects when taken in toxic doses. When they find one, they prescribe a special diluted preparation of that substance: a homeopathic remedy.

For example, it is well known that bee stings cause pain and swelling. Therefore, in order to treat various kinds of pain and swelling, a homeopath may prescribe Apis, a preparation made from bee venom. A "6x" homeopathic preparation of bee venom consists of a solution that has been diluted by a factor of ten, six times in succession. This highly dilute solution is then made into a small sugar pill that can dissolve under the tongue.

The greater the dilution, the greater the "homeopathic potency," so that a 30x solution is considered to be much stronger than a 6x. Interestingly, it is a fact of physics that a 30x homeopathic preparation contains not a single molecule of the original substance. Homeopaths believe, however, that an "energy imprint" remains when the material substance has gone.

The practice of classical homeopathy is holistic, in that it seeks to find a remedy that suits the whole person. For example, bee stings may tend to produce irritability. Therefore, a homeopathic preparation of bee venom might be prescribed to a person who suffers from irritability as well as complains of pain and swelling.

The process of matching a remedy to the whole person is lengthy and requires the services of a sophisticated homeopathic practitioner. However, homeopathy can also be used in a simplified form that focuses on particular diseases. Homeopathic remedies for such problems as flu, colds, and bladder infections are widely available in health food stores and even pharmacies. This form of treatment should probably be called symptomatic homeopathy.

WHO PRACTICES HOMEOPATHY?

Originally, homeopaths and naturopaths strongly opposed one another's methods. Homeopaths viewed herbs as allopathic, and naturopaths thought homeopathic remedies unnatural. But today homeopathy has largely been accepted into the fold of the naturopathic tradition. Naturopathic practitioners commonly prescribe herbs and homeopathics simultaneously (a combination that would have Hahnemann turning over in his grave). There are also many alternative practitioners who practice homeopathy alone.

Since there is no overall certifying body for homeopaths, each practitioner must be evaluated on an individual basis, regarding education, experience, and attitude.

HOW WELL DOES HOMEOPATHY WORK?

From a modern point of view, it is hard to believe that a few elegant principles can serve as the basis of a universal approach to treating illnesses. But Hahnemann's contemporaries had no difficulty swallowing the concept. It was the heady century following Isaac Newton, when it seemed that all nature would soon succumb to simple mathematical analysis. Newton's famous axioms (such as "For every action there is an equal but opposite reaction") had explained everything from the movements of the planets to the trajectory of cannonballs. Following his examples, intellectuals of every persuasion hoped to discover similar fundamental principles of nature.

Centuries of disillusionment later, scientists today no longer expect to find elegant rules anywhere but in physics and mathematics. The very simplicity of homeopathy's three rules now seems unrealistic.

Further arguing against homeopathy as a serious form of treatment is a fact already mentioned: homeopathic preparations contain no material elements besides the sugar used as a binder. It would be easy to dismiss homeopathy as placebo treatment but for the surprising evidence of a few research studies.

Homeopathic tablets are ideally suited for double-blind experiments. Many such studies have been carried out, and some seem to indicate that homeopathy outperforms placebos. If this is true, homeopathy must operate by some previously unrecognized force of nature.

Of course, there is always the possibility that the research on homeopathy was not performed properly. One study made it all the way to publication in the British medical journal *Lancet* before it was shown to be tainted by unconscious observer bias. Perhaps all the studies are wrong; perhaps not. A definitive statement on this subject cannot be made until more acceptable research is performed and repeated by unbiased scientists.

In my clinical experience, homeopathy sometimes seems to work, especially with children. It seems to be far less effective with adults. Many homeopaths recognize the same distinction, which they attribute to children's being more sensitive and responsive than adults. But another explanation is possible: children, being more suggestible, may respond more readily to placebo treatment. Personally, I'm not sure which is true.

SECTION III

THE HEALING ARTS

In this section I turn to those branches of alternative medicine that function more as crafts than as sciences. These methods did not originate from within the culture of Western science, nor do they depend to any significant extent on information provided by scientific research. Rather, they arose out of the pragmatic experience of a lineage of craftsmen.

Principally, I am referring to three categories of treatments: Chinese medicine, the bodywork arts (chiropractic, massage, movement therapies, and osteopathy), and the various forms of body/mind medicine.

Healing arts differ dramatically from scientific approaches to healing. Conventional medicine focuses on what can be weighed and measured, standardized and duplicated. But practitioners of the healing arts feel free to use intuitive and informal methods. Many of their techniques depend on "feel" and "gut sense." While such intangible sources of information are inadmissible in the court of science, they can be quite useful in the real world of healing.

The healing arts are warmer and fundamentally more humanizing than sciences. In a sense, they are "more alternative" than modern naturopathy. Instead of vitamins and standardized herbal extracts, so similar to the pills and tablets of conventional medicine, they make use of the invisible gifts of skilled hands and eyes.

Although they are not scientific, the best of these methods are highly pragmatic. The founders of Rolfing and Feldenkrais, for example, paid careful attention to their results and sought with all their native abilities to create methods that actually worked. They succeeded, and the healing arts that have come down through these and other traditions can be substantially effective.

Healing arts suffer from one built-in limitation, however: they are not easy to study scientifically. They are simply too fluid and subjective to fit into fully controlled experiments. For this reason it is difficult to determine exactly how effective the various healing arts are.

In scientific forms of medicine, it is much easier to weed out wishful thinking, incorrect traditions, commercialism, and ungrounded ideology; in the world of alternative medicine, all these errors and more abound. Nonetheless, mixed with the nonsense is much that is startlingly useful.

Besides the relative effectiveness of the various healing arts, within each profession there is also a wide variation in skill between practitioners. Skill in a healing art is not a commodity. To obtain good results, it is crucially important to choose an excellent practitioner. Because there is no straightforward way to do so, I devote much attention to the subject in the following chapters.

CHAPTER 6

Chinese Medicine

What we call conventional medicine is the fruit of Western scientific culture. The Eastern half of the world has its own extensive traditions of healing. These are fundamentally different from both conventional medicine and the various forms of alternative medicine originating in the West, but they are mature, comprehensive, and often highly effective.

The major Eastern healing traditions are Oriental medicine (originating in China) and Ayurveda (from India). Each of these systems is founded on ancient tradition modified over millennia of pragmatic experience. Over time they became comprehensive medical systems, possessing an extensive body of information and a systematic means of addressing all possible disease states.

(I will use the terms *Chinese medicine* and *Oriental medicine* interchangeably in this chapter. While essentially the same system is used with slight variations in many Asian countries, its Chinese origin is acknowledged by all.)

In their countries of origin, these traditions *were* the conventional approaches to medicine. This contrasts sharply with naturopathy and chiropractic, fields that originated as a rebellion against the dominance of conventional medicine. Practitioners of Eastern healing arts feel no historical rivalry with medical doctors. Secure in the embrace of a powerful and independently authoritative tradition, they look on conventional medicine more as a strong young rival than as an enemy.

One characteristic that distinguishes the Eastern medical systems from other branches of alternative medicine is their greater level of maturity. Naturopathy and chiropractic are just emerging out of the idealism of youth, when all things seem possible. (The same may be said of conventional medicine.) But these ancient Eastern approaches to healing were tempered by reality millennia ago. They have long stopped embracing simplistic theories of illness and magic cure-alls. Oriental medicine and Ayurveda are notably practical, pragmatic, and endowed with a healthy sense of their own limitations.

The philosophical basis of Eastern medicine is fundamentally different from what Westerners are used to. However, it is not necessary that a patient be Asian or subscribe to Eastern philosophies to utilize these medical traditions. Both Ayurveda and Oriental medicine are effective as techniques. Offering tools and methods that conveniently complement those of conventional medicine, they can make a substantial contribution to the health of an individual who seeks their aid.

In the United States, the most well known branch of Chinese medicine is acupuncture, but this medical system also encompasses herbology, massage (acupressure or Shiatsu), manipulation (tuina), therapeutic diet, and exercise systems such as tai chi.

There are probably at least twenty thousand practitioners of Oriental medicine in the United States. In contrast, qualified Ayurvedic physicians are rare. The situation may change in the future, as author Deepak Chopra attempts to popularize Ayurvedic techniques. But for now, in practical terms the Chinese-influenced approach is the only Eastern method most individuals can obtain. For this reason, I devote the remainder of this chapter to Chinese medicine, and leave Ayurveda to be explored by others.

THE UNIQUENESS OF CHINESE MEDICINE

When people approach a naturopathic practitioner, they encounter an approach to medicine that seems familiar. Instead of drugs, they are given herbs and supplements; rather than giving blood, they offer a sample of their hair for laboratory analysis; but essentially, the process is quite similar.

The flavor, style, and orientation of Chinese medicine are something else again. If Dorothy were in an acupuncturist's office, she might say, "Toto, now I know we're not in Kansas anymore." The expectations and mode of approach of an Oriental-style practitioner are sufficiently unusual that, without some introduction into what to expect, the new user of Chinese medical services will likely be somewhat confused. For this reason, before moving on to acupuncture and Chinese herbology, I will briefly introduce the unique Oriental approach to health and illness. Books that delve more deeply into the subject are listed in the Resources section.

Balance

The major insight and guiding principle of Chinese medicine is this: Health is a state of balance, while illness is a disturbance of that balance. All the efforts of an Oriental practitioner tend toward restoring equilibrium.

Conventional medicine tends to view illness as being caused by a single disturbance, such as a high level of cholesterol or an ovarian cyst. Treatment consists of an attempt to control or overcome this one disturbance. But in Chinese medical thought, health depends on an intricate and delicate balance of numerous factors. These must be adjusted rather than conquered.

According to Chinese medicine, the web of influences that determine health includes physical, emotional, environmental, and genetic influences. Optimum health results when these are brought into proper harmony. Few influences are seen as actually bad in themselves, but only insofar as they lead away from the equilibrium of all factors. Even emotions are to be balanced: just as there can be too much sadness, some illnesses are said to be attributable to too much joy.

This philosophy demands highly personalized medical interventions. Properly speaking, there is no such thing as an "acupuncture prescription for migraine headaches." Patients with migraines are supposed to receive unique treatment based on details of their personal condition.

Many people who encounter Chinese medicine for the first time find this highly individualized approach difficult to understand. Conventional medicine has trained them to expect health care providers to present treatments based on a named diagnosis. In the case of migraines, a medical doctor would prescribe the safest and most effective migraine medication. A naturopathic practitioner would function similarly, by recommending the herb or supplement currently most popular as a treatment for migraine.

But properly practiced Chinese medicine is never like this. Two different migraine sufferers might receive completely different treatments, based on the person, not the diagnosis. Theoretically, the treatment for one would even be expected to harm the other. Every patient requires a different intervention to push him or her toward balance. Figuratively, those who are leaning to the left need to be pushed to the right; those leaning forward, to the back. There is no one push that will put every patient aright.

I should admit that the picture I have just painted is an ideal. In real life, through the effects of human laziness, some practitioners of Oriental medicine begin to ignore the personalized approach their tradition emphasizes. They drift toward a reduced version of Oriental medicine that is more like conventional and naturopathic treatment. Instead of using the Chinese medical system to analyze each individual and determine his or her personal deficits, these "Westernized" practitioners fall back on standardized "acupuncture prescriptions." This "Westernization" of Chinese medicine debases and cheapens a tradition that has much to offer in its full and original flower.

The Holism of Oriental Medicine

Another dramatic difference between Chinese medical thought and the approach taken by conventional medicine is the former's remarkable holism. Whereas medicine in the West tends to focus its attention on minute details and consider them in isolation from the rest of the body, the Oriental approach takes the person as a whole. This follows from the basic Oriental philosophy that illness is due to lack of balance. Obviously, it is impossible to restore balance by looking only at details; the big picture is essential.

According to Chinese thought, body, mind, and spirit are inextricably woven together into a single fabric of life. This can be seen clearly in the traditional set of questions Oriental practitioners ask at the beginning of an office visit. Factors that are connected in the practitioner's mind often seem strikingly unrelated to Western ears.

For example, if a patient complains of gallbladder pain, an Oriental physician would ask many of the same questions as an M.D. "Do you get right-sided abdominal pain in the middle of the night?" is just as pertinent for both professionals. But only the Oriental doctor would follow this up by asking "Do you have an explosive temper?" and "Do you have trouble arriving at decisions?" In the holistic viewpoint of Oriental medicine, emotional characteristics such as these might be important details to distinguish between various gallbladder imbalances.

This interweaving of various levels often surprises those who are used to the more compartmentalized style of Western medicine. I remember the wide-eyed look a patient with a bad cough gave me when I asked her whether she had just suffered some grief. "Are you psychic?" she asked, astounded. "No," I replied, "but Chinese medicine links the lungs with sadness." It turned out that her mother had just died.

The holism of Chinese medical theory can be amazing, but there is always a difference between intentions and results. Even though Chinese medicine intends to address the whole being, it does not always do so successfully, or in the best way possible. The theory doesn't always work as well as advertised.

Too many acupuncturists graduate from school with the mistaken belief that a rigid application of the system they have learned will always work. According to this idealized view, practically everyone can be healed of all their illnesses simply by paying for enough acupuncture treatments. Even if a given patient does not seem to get better, the acupuncturist may say to himself, "I'm sure it did him some good at a deep level," and keep on applying the technique tradition teaches.

This is a problem essentially opposite to the Westernization of Chinese medicine just described. While that trend leads to a disregarding of all traditional theory, the acupuncturist who is too certain of her or his concepts makes the reverse error. A theory is only an approximation of the truth. The successful practice of any form of medicine involves a pragmatic ability to respond to results. Good acupuncturists are flexible.

Naming Illnesses

Besides the concept of balance and the drive toward holism, Chinese medicine differs from conventional medicine in another feature: It uses a completely different method of naming illnesses than what we are familiar with in the West. This fundamental distinction often causes confusion.

Western medicine tends to organize diseases around causes. Thus a child may develop "strep throat," named after the streptococcal bacteria that are flourishing in such infections. Or the child may come down with "insulin-dependent diabetes," so named because the disease is caused by a lack of insulin.

Because we are familiar with this way of naming illnesses, it seems the only possible way. But it isn't. These names are not descriptions of absolute realities but only arbitrary shorthand expressions. No two people with strep throat are actually sick in exactly the same way, nor are two cases of diabetes alike. However, since it would be impossible to give every single form of an illness its own name, conventional medicine uses terms like *strep throat* for convenience.

Oriental medicine has also developed categories of illness to bring order out of chaos, but they are constructed differently. Chinese medical thought pays less attention to causes than to overall patterns.

For example, consider two patients who are sneezing. Let us say that one has a cold and the other suffers from sinus allergies. These are two different Western diagnoses, distinguished because the first is caused by a virus, the second by an immune dysfunction. However, both patients might be diagnosed with a single Oriental diagnosis. The symptom pattern of cough, sinus congestion, and fatigue suggests the syndrome named "superficial invasion of wind-cold." In this example, two different Western medical diagnoses fall under one broad Oriental one.

But it can go the other way too. Two patients with the medical diagnosis of asthma might fit into one of at least five different Oriental patterns. Which one would depend on the answers to such questions as, "Do you feel shorter of breath on exhalation or on inhalation? Are your lungs dry or phlegmy? Is your digestion good? Are your hands and feet often cold?" Medical doctors make nothing of such distinctions. To them, asthma is asthma. But to an Oriental practitioner various answers to these questions might indicate completely different approaches to treatment.

Neither system of diagnosing is more correct or less correct; the two techniques simply represent different ways to organize the complex realm of human sickness. One slices the cake up and down, the other side to side. Actually, there are billions of ways to be sick, and only a few thousand names of illnesses. Every system of naming is just a simplification for convenience' sake.

The availability of an alternative system of naming can be a great boon for at least one category of patients: those who suffer from symptoms that conventional medicine cannot identify. There are many such people, and nearly every one of them is frustrated and despondent over the inability of their medical doctors to give their symptoms a name. Oriental medicine can sometimes help.

I remember Darlene, a patient who suffered from a seemingly strange collection of symptoms. Darlene first visited her doctor to evaluate the lump she felt in her throat while swallowing. He sent her to an ear, nose, and throat specialist, but the ENT found nothing. Subsequently, she began to feel slightly nauseated all the time, coupled with a constant urge to burp. A gastroenterologist (digestion specialist) looked at her, but he too could not identify the presence of any disease.

Next Darlene lost her appetite, and her abdomen began to swell. Her worried primary care doctor sent her back to the gastroenterologist, who subjected her to many intrusive and unpleasant tests. The results yielded nothing.

Over the next several months, Darlene's menstrual periods became irregular and painful, and she complained of intense PMS symptoms. Again she visited doctors of several varieties, and again none could find anything wrong.

Obviously, Darlene was not well. But according to her doctors, she was not sick. They began to assume that she was either depressed, a hypochondriac, or a fake. Her friends, relatives, and employers started to take the same attitude, as each test and exam came back negative.

But Darlene was sick. It was just that her particular sickness didn't have a name in conventional medicine. If her symptoms had fit a known problem, her doctors would have probably known what to do to help her. But the symptoms didn't fit, and so the doctors could do nothing.

Being sick is bad enough. When no one believes you're sick, you begin to feel crazy as well. The whole experience finally did make Darlene depressed. She was just about to ask for an antidepressant when good fortune surprised her with a solution to her problems. At a party, Darlene happened to meet an acupuncturist. Some impulse drove her to retell her whole sad story. Darlene expected the acupuncturist to cluck and then politely excuse herself, but she didn't. Instead, the acupuncturist listened attentively, and at the end remarked, "If I didn't know better, I would think you'd been reading textbooks of Chinese medicine. You have the most classic example of a famous Oriental diagnosis I have ever seen outside of a book."

Darlene's symptoms, so peculiar and unrelated according to Western medicine, fitted precisely into the classic textbook description of "stagnant liver Qi." This is a rather common Oriental diagnosis, as common in the East as migraine headaches or hypertension is in the West. Darlene was a more full-blown case of it than most. The average person diagnosed with "stagnant liver Qi" manifests only a few of the symptoms; Darlene demonstrated practically every one. A first-year acupuncture student would have recognized the signs, but no medical doctor could. The syndrome simply does not exist in conventional medicine.

Because she could easily identify Darlene's disease in the Oriental system of medicine, the acupuncturist could easily devise a treatment for her. Darlene had been sick for over a year. It took only one month of acupuncture and Chinese herbs to restore Darlene to health.

I frequently meet patients whose symptoms do not fit any conventional diagnosis. It isn't rare. Although it is a surprisingly little known fact, conventional medicine does not have a name for every problem. Sometimes the Oriental approach discovers an identifiable illness where a medical doctor sees only unrelated and inexplicable symptoms.

I do not mean to imply by this that Oriental medicine is better at making diagnoses than conventional medicine. The two systems are merely different. However, this difference represents a great opportunity for those patients who have exhausted the resources of conventional medicine. They have the option of an entirely fresh approach.

Having described some of the unique characteristics of Chinese medical thought, I will now turn to the two major forms of Chinese treatment available in this country: acupuncture and Chinese herbology. Shiatsu (acupressure) is discussed in the following chapter under the heading of massage.

ACUPUNCTURE

Although acupuncture is many thousands of years old, it has only become popular in this country since the middle 1970s. American awareness of acupuncture developed after President Nixon traveled to China. One of his aides had developed acute appendicitis, and rather than being flown out of the country he was operated on by a Chinese team. What caught everyone's attention was that the surgery was performed using acupuncture for anesthesia. The event triggered an explosion of American interest in this traditional Chinese art.

At the present time, there are about forty colleges of acupuncture in the United States. Twenty-nine states license acupuncturists, and there are a total of about ten thousand licensed acupuncturists practicing nationwide. An unknown number of additional acupuncturists practice underground in states where there is no licensure available. Finally, many chiropractors and medical doctors practice a form of acupuncture within the scope of their general licenses.

Acupuncture is still in its infancy as a profession in America. Educational requirements for licensure vary from state to state, and in some states the practice of acupuncture is still essentially illegal. A National Commission for the Certification of Acupuncturists (the NCCA) exists, but not all states that issue licenses use its standard certifying test. The American Association of Acupuncture and Oriental Medicine (AAAOM) is acupuncture's equivalent of the AMA, but its membership includes only one-fifth of the total number of licensed acupuncturists in practice.

Because it is so young in the United States, acupuncture is one of the most rapidly growing of all health professions. It tends to attract students who are sincere, idealistic, and intellectually sophisticated. The field offers a tremendous potential for career growth, as there are few areas in the country where the market for acupuncturists is saturated.

Relations between acupuncturists and M.D.s are among the best in all of alternative medicine, for a variety of reasons. In contrast to naturopathy and chiropractic, acupuncture is not a traditional rival of conventional medicine. Therefore, there is no bad blood to overcome. Also, some medical doctors use a treatment method somewhat similar to acupuncture themselves, called trigger-point therapy. This gives them a sense of familiarity with acupuncture. Finally, the evidence of acupuncture anesthesia viscerally impresses doctors, who conclude that the treatment must be effective if it can overcome the pain of surgery.

In some states, governmental agencies employ acupuncturists for their aid in drug detoxification programs. Numerous insurance policies reimburse acupuncture, although often only when it is an M.D. who practices it. This distinction rankles licensed acupuncturists, who point out that while they must complete thousands of hours of training in acupuncture as part of the requirements for their licensure, in almost all states M.D.s are allowed to practice acupuncture with no special training.

What Is Acupuncture Good For?

Acupuncture is most well known as a treatment for chronic pain conditions. These include musculoskeletal problems such as neck pain and back pain, as well as nerve-related pain and pain problems of a more internal nature. Table 5-1 rates the effectiveness of acupuncture by pain condition. Please note that these ratings are based on my clinical impression. Not enough good studies have been performed to make a truly objective evaluation possible.

Table 5-1

Effectiveness of acupuncture for pain conditions.

Condition	Effectiveness
Musculoskeletal Pain	
Arthritis	Moderate
Acute back pain	Excellent
Chronic low-back pain	Moderate
Fibromyalgia	Poor to Moderate
Whiplash injury	Excellent (especially certain Japanese forms of acupuncture)
Chronic neck pain	Moderate
Plantar fasciitis	Moderate
Tendinitis	Moderate
Tension headaches	Excellent
Nerve-related Pain	
Carpal tunnel syndrome	Poor to Moderate
Morton's neuroma	Poor to Moderate
Peripheral neuropathy	Poor to Excellent
Thoracic outlet syndrome	Poor to Moderate
Other Forms of Pain	
Dysmenorrhea	Moderate to Excellent
Irritable bowel syndrome	Moderate to Excellent
Migraine headaches	Poor to Excellent
Sinus headaches	Moderate

Success with these (and all other) conditions depends to a large extent on the skill of the acupuncturist, the particular type of acupuncture used, and, of course, the severity of the problem. Previous surgery in an area tends to make acupuncture for pain in that area less successful.

Besides pain, acupuncture can also be used for a wide variety of other conditions. In Asia acupuncture is traditionally considered to be a complete system of medical care. The theory of acupuncture is broad and flexible enough to approach every possible health problem.

Of course, theory and reality are two distinct subjects. I personally do not believe that acupuncture is as universally powerful as its proponents maintain. Nonetheless, I have frequently seen acupuncture treat internal medicine conditions successfully. There are too many possible examples to list them all, but the following gives some idea of acupuncture's potential scope: Acupuncture can sometimes shrink the size of uterine fibroids, markedly diminish the symptoms of asthma, break the cycle of recurrent sinus infections, relieve depression and anxiety, lower elevated blood pressure, provoke remissions in cases of rheumatoid arthritis, and reduce insulin requirements in adult-onset diabetics.

Acupuncture certainly does not always succeed with the conditions just described. My general impression is that superior acupuncturists can alleviate internal medical problems at a rate that is significantly greater than can be accounted for by placebo, but less than 70 percent. On the other hand, mediocre acupuncturists seldom succeed with any health problems other than pain.

Finally, acupuncture is commonly represented as being able to prevent illnesses, but I have been unimpressed with the results. In my experience, patients undergoing regular acupuncture still get sick. Perhaps acupuncture treatment makes such problems less frequent, but, if so, the effect must be subtle. Prevention probably depends more on the lifestyle of the patient than on intervention by a physician, of whatever persuasion.

How Quickly Does Acupuncture Work?

Often the effects of acupuncture are not immediate. A patient may go home from a treatment continuing to hurt, and may not notice any improvement until the next day or after several treatments. When acupuncture finally begins to work, however, the effects can be prolonged, continuing weeks, months, or years after the treatment is stopped.

For most chronic pain conditions, six sessions should be enough to show if the treatment is going to work. It is not that those six sessions should produce a complete cure, but there should be some response at that point to justify further treatment. This response may involve no more than a brief lightening of symptoms or a change of symptom patterns. Such a sign indicates that the acupuncture is managing to affect the problem.

If there is no change at all after six treatments, chances are that continued treatments will produce no results. When there are encouraging indications, treatment should be continued until maximum benefit is reached. Initial treatments may be performed at intervals of once or twice a week. The number of sessions should gradually taper off as symptoms improve and then finally stop altogether.

Acupuncture pain treatment tends to be synergistic with chiropractic. It is probably fair to say that one treatment of each is better than two of either one alone.

For conditions other than pain, acupuncture may take much longer to produce its effect. Three months of weekly treatments should be long enough to give an indication whether there is any hope of benefit.

These recommendations are just rules of thumb. Every individual is different. I remember a patient, whom I shall call Joan, who had suffered from severe migraines twice weekly for forty years. On my advice she sought the services of an acupuncturist. After listening to her story, the practitioner expressed some reservations. He did not want to raise her expectations too high because, as he explained, problems that have endured over ten years are always very difficult to treat. Joan felt momentarily dismayed, but then bounced back. She felt a strong inner inclination to try acupuncture.

After six sessions nothing had changed. The migraines still came on schedule, with no noticeable alteration in severity, timing, or quality. Discouraged, the acupuncturist was ready to quit, but Joan insisted on continuing. Again, at twenty sessions the practitioner wanted to stop, but again she overruled him. Driven by Joan's tenacity, but against his professional instincts, the acupuncturist continued to treat her for nine fruitless months. Finally, Joan too abandoned hope, and stopped coming. Two weeks after she terminated treatment her headaches stopped, and never returned.

I don't know why it worked this way. Most people who do not respond in the first several sessions will never respond. I would never have encouraged Joan to keep trying that long; I would regard the acupuncturist as a sleazy salesman if he had kept her coming in on his own initiative. But Joan felt an intuition to continue, and it proved correct.

Cases like Joan's encourage some acupuncturists to treat all patients indefinitely in hopes of an eventual cure. However, there is a law of diminishing returns in alternative medicine as elsewhere. The chances of recovery decrease with the number of ineffective treatments. Most responsible acupuncturists will soon quit if they "cannot touch the symptom."

Because one acupuncturist fails, however, does not mean that acupuncture itself is useless. Some acupuncturists are much better than others, and there are many different styles and methods. I have often seen another acupuncturist succeed where one or more have given up.

How Does Acupuncture Work?

The only honest answer to this question is: no one knows. Acupuncture was born during the Bronze Age of ancient China. No one then cared to ask how it worked. What concerned ancient doctors was only "What can we do to make this method work even better?"

In the West, we are used to seeking explanations for results, because discovering how things work has been the special fascination of our culture for the last half-millennium. But such a quest for explanation is not universal. Nor is it essential for developing and refining useful techniques.

Ming dynasty ceramic artists could not have explained the chemistry behind their glazes, but that didn't stop them from producing glazed pottery of surpassing excellence. Closer to home, medical researchers have repeatedly discovered powerful drugs by accident, and brought them to market even though their method of function remains unknown. Results do not depend on answering the question, "How does this work?"

Only in the last two decades have Western investigators begun to look for acupuncture's mechanism of action. The first studies quickly demonstrated that it was not going to be an easy problem to solve.

For example, acupuncture theory describes twelve "lines of energy" on the body, which it calls "meridians." Nearly all the acupuncture points lie on these meridians, and acupuncture treatment commonly involves the treatment of points at one end of a meridian to produce effects at the other end. The meridian lines do not match the pattern of the nervous system very closely. Early researchers tried to find undiscovered physical structures in the body that would match the meridians as classically described, but they did not succeed. Whatever the meridians may be, they are not visible under the microscope. Nonetheless, treatment at one end of a meridian does sometimes produce obvious effects further down the line.

Subsequent studies provided some information that was interesting, if not definitive. They showed that acupuncture causes a release of endorphins, the now-famous naturally occurring morphinelike substances. Furthermore, they demonstrated that needling produces changes in the electrical conductivity of the skin. But whether these observations are important or incidental remains unclear.

Many authors blithely explain acupuncture in terms of indirect nerve stimulation, endorphin release, or skin resistance changes, but these explanations are really no more than entertaining speculations. The available information on acupuncture is so fragmentary and incomplete that to theorize about how acupuncture works is simply to wag one's tongue. No one really knows enough about it to draw any conclusions.

Perhaps future work will discover the biological mechanisms underlying acupuncture. Unfortunately, there simply is not a lot of money available for basic acupuncture research. Some funding is supporting studies to evaluate how well acupuncture works, a different subject entirely.

How Well Does Acupuncture Work?

Acupuncturists tend to believe that their technique must be effective because it has endured so long. While there is certainly good sense in this presumption, traditional use is not an entirely reliable guide. Many ineffective practices have survived the test of time, at least so far as belief in them goes.

But acupuncturists have a history of being conspicuously pragmatic and realistic about the application of their craft. They have evaluated their treatments and courageously abandoned methods that didn't work. Because of this tradition of pragmatism, it is reasonable to expect that much of acupuncture is truly useful. However, it is also more than likely that some aspects of acupuncture are completely wrong.

The only solid way to determine the effectiveness of a craft like acupuncture is through systematic studies. These are difficult to perform, however, for three reasons: First, the highly individualized nature of acupuncture makes it hard to design standardized tests. Second, sources of funding for acupuncture research are few. There is no deep-pocket equivalent of pharmaceutical companies in the field of acupuncture, and other sources of money tend to flow toward "sexier" high-tech subjects. Finally, the people most skilled at research and possessing access to funding are not usually the same as those with a high level of understanding of acupuncture theory and practice.

Studies performed in China have tended to concentrate on comparing one acupuncture approach to another, rather than on evaluating the effectiveness of acupuncture per se. Fortunately, despite many obstacles, a number of intriguing acupuncture research studies have been performed in the West.

Research has demonstrated that acupuncture can be effective for dental pain, headaches, low-back pain, neck pain, tennis elbow, dysmenorrhea, asthma, recovery from strokes, nausea, and insomnia. For funding reasons, nearly all these studies involved thirty or fewer patients. The results were strong enough to give a definite indication that acupuncture can work. Much more research must still be done to provide a solid scientific basis for acupuncture as an effective treatment.

It is my clinical impression that the success rate of acupuncture appears to be among the highest of all the alternative medical options, and for many individuals its results compare favorably with conventional options. But I have observed a strange phenomenon regarding the success or failure of acupuncture. It seems that if a person responds to acupuncture for one complaint, he or she will most likely have a positive result with another ailment as well. Conversely, if acupuncture has failed to treat a person's frozen shoulder, a sinus infection will not respond either. I cannot explain why this happens, nor predict who will respond. It is as if some people have the word "acupuncture me" written on their foreheads in invisible ink. Unlike placebo treatments, this susceptibility to cure does not seem to depend on belief. I have often seen nonbelievers cured and believers walk away sick.

Why acupuncture (or any other healing art) will cure one person and fail to help another remains enigmatic. The key either fits the lock, or it doesn't. This mystery troubles me. I wish there were a way to know in advance whether acupuncture, chiropractic, or another approach will prove successful. Such foreknowledge would help avoid expensive and frustrating processes of trial and error. Yet I know of no shortcut to determine in advance which healing art (if any) will work for a particular individual.

What to Expect During a Visit

Most acupuncturists work on their own, without a receptionist or nurses. The office is typically informally decorated, without the luxury sometimes seen in chiropractors' offices and private medical clinics. Usually some signs of Oriental culture are visible, such as prints or artifacts, and there is a sense communicated of long Asian tradition.

Each session begins with the acupuncturist asking a series of questions covering physical, emotional, and environmental conditions. Then the practitioner examines the patient's tongue, takes the pulse in a characteristically detailed fashion, and often palpates the abdomen. These aspects of the physical examination have specific meanings in Chinese medicine. For example, a white tongue coating may indicate the presence of a pattern known as "damp spleen." This pattern might be confirmed by puffiness above the navel and a pulse that feels rounded and full.

After formulating a plan, the acupuncturist then begins treatment. This primarily involves inserting disposable needles into specific locations known as acupuncture points. The needles may be inserted very superficially, or to a depth of one or more inches, depending on the particular point and the style of treatment being used. Sometimes the points are also stimulated with heat or electricity. Acupuncture needles are typically retained for twenty to forty minutes.

Acupuncturists may also prescribe Chinese herbal combinations and possibly give dietary advice. They do not make medical diagnoses or speculate on medical causes of symptoms, nor do they give naturopathic advice. While acupuncture shares some concepts in common with naturopathy, the two approaches are too different to be easily melded. Therefore, there usually is no point in asking an acupuncturist for advice on vitamins and food supplements.

Dangers of Acupuncture

Acupuncture is quite safe. Occasionally it can produce a temporary flare-up of symptoms, but these are almost always limited to no more than a few days. Small bruises are common too.

Serious consequences of acupuncture are rare. Because the needles used are disposable, there is no risk of AIDS or hepatitis. An incautious acupuncturist can puncture the lung or other vital organ, or produce bleeding by piercing a large blood vessel. Patients who take blood thinners such as coumadin (warfarin) should probably not get acupuncture, due to the increased risk of internal bleeding.

Alternative practitioners are often accused of keeping their patients away from necessary medical treatment. However, this is seldom the case with acupuncturists, who are almost always respectful of conventional medicine. They may encourage their patients to consider reducing their medications, but only when their symptoms decrease and under medical supervision. This compatibility may be attributed to the fact that a model already exists for cooperation between Oriental and Western approaches in China, where the two are typically used concurrently.

As with all forms of alternative medicine, the main danger in acupuncture treatment is the risk that it may fail.

Identifying an Excellent Acupuncturist

Much more so than with medical doctors, the choice of acupuncturist is absolutely crucial. Medical doctors depend primarily on their mastery of a body of certified knowledge. It is the quality of established medical information that matters most. Personal gifts are secondary. Naturopathic practitioners function in much the same way.

But acupuncturists, like all craftspeople, rely to a great extent on personal skills and talents. Practitioners are definitely not interchangeable. The range of competency from the best to the worst is immense in every craft, and acupuncture is no exception.

Of course, acupuncturists don't label themselves as "mediocre" or "just beginning." They may recite their credentials, such as "trained in China" or "certified by the National Board," but such résumé items say little about actual skill. No specific criteria can determine who is a good acupuncturist.

The situation is further complicated by the fact that acupuncture in the United States is very diverse. There are many distinct styles of acupuncture, including TCM (traditional Chinese medicine), Japanese Manaka style, Korean hand acupuncture, ear acupuncture, and the Worsley method. Advocates of each field tend to believe that their method is better than all others. The situation is so complex that to have tried acupuncture with several practitioners is not necessarily to have received all that acupuncture has to offer.

As a bare minimum, an acupuncturist should be licensed by the state in which she or he practices, if such a license exists. If there is no license available, the practitioner should have graduated from an accredited acupuncture school (see the accreditation commissions information in the Resources section) or otherwise satisfied the requirements of the National Commission for the Certification of Acupuncturists. Beyond verifying these credentials, identifying well-qualified acupuncturists is a judgment call. Getting a recommendation from someone with expertise in the field is the best option.

Acupuncturists to be avoided come in two kinds: those who attempt to use acupuncture as a purely technical method without any interest in theory or philosophy; and those on the other extreme who have fallen in love with the ideals and theories of acupuncture and have lost touch with reality.

In the former category belong most medical doctors and chiropractors who perform acupuncture. The great majority of these ignore theory entirely, and use an extremely simplified version of acupuncture. A leading exponent of this approach is the medical doctor George Ulett. In his book *Beyond Yin and Yang*, Dr. Ulett dismisses the entire tradition of acupuncture as fanciful metaphysics and numerology. He proposes that medical doctors can learn acupuncture without any reference to the tradition. This approach does not do justice to the craft of acupuncture.

At the other extreme are acupuncturists who follow theory slavishly and pay no attention to results. New graduates of acupuncture school are most likely to exhibit these symptoms, along with practitioners of the more idealistic schools of acupuncture, such as the Worsley method.

The best acupuncturists achieve a balance between pragmatism and theoretical understanding. Although I am not certain of the exact count, I believe that I have personally received treatment from at least thirty acupuncturists. In order to help you identify superior practitioners, I will profile three types of acupuncturists, based on actual people I have known.

The first acupuncturist is a medical doctor who has practiced a simplified form of acupuncture for ten years. The second is an overly idealistic acupuncturist. The third is an example of a sophisticated and balanced practitioner. I present them as if they were describing themselves.

Profile of a Westernized Acupuncturist

Scott Randolph, M.D.: I first trained with Dr. Joseph Helms (a prominent and highly regarded educator of M.D. acupuncturists) at his intensive three-month course in Los Angeles. For years I practiced just as he taught us to do, with all that yin and yang, sun and moon stuff. But after a while I started to discard the ethnic colors. I came to believe that acupuncture is simply a technique; that all the philosophical ideas historically associated with it are just excess baggage.

The theory behind acupuncture is typical of medieval thinking. For example, traditional acupuncturists believe that every part of the body corresponds to the whole, whether it's the ear or the bottom of the foot. But that's just sympathetic magic. It's voodoo. The real world doesn't operate that way.

Acupuncture works by affecting the electrical resistance of the skin. You see, when you use an instrument that can measure the electrical conductivity of the skin, you discover that the acupuncture points are sites of lowered resistance. When the needles are stimulated, a reversal occurs, and the same areas become regions of high resistance.

I don't know how the ancient Chinese stumbled on this effect. The theory they invented to explain it is archaic and fantastical, but the technique of needle insertion really works.

When a patient has back or neck pain, acupuncture can provide dramatic relief, far more than drugs or physical therapy. I insert the needles in the right locations and twist and turn them gently. Waves of relaxation move through the body. Pain diminishes rapidly, and often permanently.

Acupuncture isn't difficult. You don't even need to study point locations. A simple twenty-dollar machine can locate the areas of lower resistance. You just stick needles in those spots, twist them a bit, and the patient begins to feel better. It's that easy.

Profile of an Excessively Idealistic Acupuncturist

Chad Sanders: Dr. Randolph isn't even doing acupuncture. He's caught up in a purely Western outlook. He does not understand—probably cannot understand—that acupuncture is rooted in a totally different paradigm. It is an Eastern school of medicine, founded on a wholly Eastern worldview.

I suppose it is interesting to know that acupuncture points have some relationship with electrical skin resistance, but it doesn't really matter. Acupuncture is not about skin resistance. It's about the movement and balancing of pure life energy.

Acupuncture, when performed properly, balances the entire body. The body is composed of five elements, or phases of energy. When any one predominates, or is deficient, the general health of a person diminishes.

As a traditional acupuncture practitioner, I set about determining which energies are out of balance. I obtain this information by taking the patient's pulse. If you really pay attention to the pulse, you will begin to notice very subtle gradations of sensations. The pulse isn't just fast or slow, weak or strong. There are thousands of possible kinds of pulses. The pulse can feel like a little ball-bearing moving under your finger, or a dab of glue. It can be firm, even hard, or soft and squishy. Some pulses seem to give way with pressure, like a drinking straw that collapses. Others feel like the taut head of a drum.

The ancient Chinese masters of healing discovered that by taking the pulse at different positions along the wrist they could determine the state of each internal organ. Because we feel for the pulse in more than one location, we acupuncturists use the plural noun form, pulses. The goal of acupuncture is to balance the pulses. When the pulses are balanced, the body is balanced and healing occurs spontaneously.

I do not even ask my patients about their symptoms. Sneezing and wheezing, coughing and aching, it doesn't matter. I can figure out everything I need to know by taking the pulse. I concentrate deeply, listening to every nuance. In time, I come to understand the essence of the person's health problems and know just what to do.

Sometimes it takes a number of treatments, but, sooner or later, acupuncture brings about complete healing. Not just a quick fix, but a full and complete restoration of health. This is the goal of acupuncture.

Profile of a Mature Practitioner

Eileen Simpson: I practice a mixture of acupuncture styles. Over the last four years I have been very influenced by Japanese techniques, particularly the work of Kiiko Matsumoto. What I have learned from Kiiko is an attitude of checking what works.

I use many techniques for diagnosis—pulse, tongue, abdomen, symptoms, and medical history. Then I try to develop a strategy based on either the traditional Chinese medical analysis or one of the modern Japanese approaches. But I always remember that I must be willing to change my plan based on results.

Kiiko likes to get feedback from the body. She trusts the body and trusts the feedback she gets. For example, suppose a patient has a lot of tension around the neck. Kiiko might use a distal point on the forearm to open up the neck area. (A distal point is a related acupuncture point some distance away from the area being treated.) Before inserting a needle, she'll work the point with her finger for a while to see if she can get a release of the target area. If she can't, she'll try a different angle, a slightly different location, or a completely different point.

When she finally finds the optimal angle and location, Kiiko then inserts a needle in precisely the place she's discovered. It's not like putting candles in a birthday cake. There's a subtle internal sensation when the needle is placed properly. The point opens up, it lets go, the Qi moves. Like Kiiko says, you can feel it with your fingers and in your own body.

I use acupuncture for a wide variety of conditions, from simple neck pain to difficult internal problems such as gallbladder disease and hypothyroidism. Although I don't always succeed, my work is getting more effective every year.

I'm always studying. I especially appreciate learning from people who have tried to adapt the traditions of acupuncture to modern situations. Don't throw away the traditions—adapt them. Acupuncture should be a constantly evolving art, respectful of tradition but flexible and open to change.

Commentary: Given a choice between these three acupuncturists, I would strongly recommend Eileen Simpson. Dr. Randolph is too limited. What he performs is so oversimplified it shouldn't really be called acupuncture. The type of acupuncture Chad Sanders practices is an example of the opposite error. Although it is based on genuine Oriental traditions, it is too dreamily idealistic. It is like an exotic hothouse flower, beautiful to look at, but too ethereal to function in the real world.

"Bratman's Rule" states that the deeper the intended level of healing, the greater the likelihood of falling off the deep end into fantasy. Only a well-grounded individual can use subtle principles successfully. Eileen has such personal integrity. She is both pragmatic and sensitive. Working like a craftsperson, she picks up clues from the whole person of the patient. Her abilities to receive feedback are well developed. Although Eileen is deeply committed to tradition, she is also open to innovations.

It is difficult to find practitioners who function at this level of competence. Perhaps only one in twenty is so gifted. Even simplistic acupuncture can do some good. But for difficult problems, it is necessary to find a highly qualified practitioner, like Eileen.

CHINESE HERBAL MEDICINE

While it can be difficult to identify the most qualified acupuncturists, at least they exist in some numbers. But there are relatively few sophisticated practitioners of Chinese herbal medicine in the United States. Oriental herbology is far more complex than the Western herbal tradition, which uses herbs like drugs to treat specific diseases and symptoms. Chinese herbs are prescribed to promote balance according to the complex principles of Chinese medicine.

Chinese herbology is a difficult academic pursuit. Herbs are organized by their effects on the energies of the body: whether they act to warm or cool, concentrate or disperse, strengthen or drain, dry or moisten, calm or activate, lubricate or bind, treat the interior or exterior, or cause energy to ascend or descend. Each herb is further thought to carry its effects primarily to specific organs or "energy layers."

Chinese herbs are seldom used alone. They are ordinarily arranged in complex compositions involving "ministerial," "deputy," "assistant," and "envoy" herbs. A Chinese herbalist analyzes the "energetics" of a patient and prescribes herbal formulas strategically designed to correct whatever imbalances may be found. The formula is changed as the patient's condition progresses.

To understand the difference between Western and Oriental herbal treatment, consider the case of a patient who presents with migraine headaches. A Western herbalist might simply prescribe feverfew, because headaches are feverfew's primary indication. In contrast, a Chinese herbalist would need to know every detail of the patient's health history. Only then would the herbalist choose a strategy of treatment.

The Chinese herbalist might discover that the migraine headaches were related to "imbalances in the liver energy." If so, she would prescribe herbs to balance the liver in the precise way it needed to be balanced according to theory. This might include increasing the energy of certain organs and dispersing the energy of others, in order to move the liver into a balanced web of right relationships with the rest of the body.

However, not all migraine headaches resolve into "liver imbalances." Some may fit a different classical description, such as "exogenous wind cold" or "gall-bladder/stomach disharmony." Every possible Oriental analysis would call for its own herbal strategy, both in the short and the long term.

This approach to treatment is obviously far more holistic than that used by Western herbalists. In Western herbology, feverfew fits all migraine headaches; the Oriental approach tailors the herbal combination to the person, not the disease.

Chinese herbology is so difficult an intellectual pursuit that only doctors of considerable scholarship can practice it skillfully. Its practice requires a kind of deep pattern recognition, an ability to see through superficial details into the underlying structure of a problem. Simultaneously, an herbalist must possess a finely developed clinical sense and considerable interpersonal skills. I am deeply impressed by the one famous herbalist I have come to know well, a woman whom I shall call Dr. Chan.

When I first met her Dr. Chan was seventy-five, although she looked no more than fifty. She had settled in San Francisco after escaping from mainland China. Dr. Chan carries herself with the gently amused dignity characteristic of many Oriental healers. Although she exudes compassion, she always remains detached and self-contained.

So knowledgeable is she regarding the nature of herbs, Dr. Chan can add new herbs to the pharmacopoeia on her own initiative. That is to say, by touching, smelling, tasting, and examining a plant unknown to Chinese tradition, she can assign it a place in that tradition and substitute it for less easily available Asian imports.

I have seen Dr. Chan produce cures or remissions in cases of dreadfully difficult diseases, such as chronic hepatitis B and C, multiple sclerosis, and rheumatoid arthritis. Lesser illnesses frequently respond to her approach quite easily. Despite her mastery of herbal treatment, however, initial tactics often fail. She frequently has to change strategies midstream several times in order to finally succeed. From time to time she gives up entirely. When necessary, Dr. Chan admits defeat graciously, explaining, "I am just learning to practice herbal medicine."

Dr. Chan does not dispense her own herbs. She writes out a fresh prescription each visit in beautiful Chinese script. This is to be taken to a traditional herbal pharmacy.

How Chinese Herbs Are Prepared

Not only is Chinese herbology vastly more complex than its equivalent in American culture, Chinese herb stores are far more entertaining. My favorite stands at a busy intersection in San Francisco's Chinatown, where the nearest parking may be twelve blocks away. The place is the size of a small warehouse, stocked to the ceiling with raw herbal supplies and packaged Chinese teas.

The most interesting ingredients stand in jars on the counter: snakeskins, antelope horn, grasshoppers, and dried worms. Like its European cousin, Chinese herbology has always included certain carefully selected animal products, although not always with the blessing of the academics.

The herb preparers use ancient counterweights to measure precise quantities of prescribed herbs in handheld balance scales. Some herbs must be roasted in honey before dispensing, a process carried out in large gas-fired woks set on the floor. Other herbs are ground up in brass mortars with pestles that ring loudly against the sides.

When it is finally ready, a formula is wrapped in white paper packets. Three packets last six days, good for one week and a recommended off-day. The ingredients consist of colorful stems, seeds, and sliced roots. These are to be boiled three times in a ceramic pot; each time the water is poured off and saved. Smelling rather reminiscent of cat urine, no Western medicine has ever tasted worse. Honey or sugar are far too weak to alter the impact. In recognition of this fact, some herb stores provide candies with the herbs, to be taken afterward as an aid in recovery from the taste of the treatment.

When I became known as a regular of this establishment and a client of Dr. Chan's, I no longer needed to find a parking place. An elderly woman would catch sight of me when I slowed to a stop by the curb, wave her hand, and flash a warm smile. She would take my prescription from the car window and indicate how long I should wait to return to the curb. At the appointed time, she would reemerge from the store to sell it to me, with much enthusiasm and dispatch.

Higher and Lower Forms of Chinese Herbology

Dr. Chan was a recognized master, but not every self-proclaimed Chinese herbalist can say as much. This art is far more difficult to learn than Western herbology.

Many practitioners of Chinese herbal medicine use a simplified form developed in Japan, known as the Kanpo system. This method of treatment is respectable, if less than ideal, and can also produce good results. The Kanpo system involves several hundred fixed herbal combinations. Although not as individualizable as the classic method, it is still flexible enough to treat a wide variety of patterns. Kanpo herbs have the additional advantage of being sold as powders that do not need to be boiled.

Chinese-made precompounded patent medicines are typically more symptomatic in their orientation, and as such considerably less than ideal. Generally, if a practitioner recommends Chinese herbs "for asthma," or "for menstrual pain," he or she is not practicing a very high form of the art. Similarly, herbalists of the Western tradition sometimes mix a few Chinese herbs into their formulas for specific conditions. Some of the most popular are ginseng, tang kuei, fo ti, mahuang, and astragalus. Such herbalists have ignored the unique holism of Chinese herbal medicine, and are prescribing these materials essentially as if they were symptomatic Western herbs. This Westernization of the art of Chinese herbology is unfortunate, but it is not the lowest form of Chinese herbology available.

The ultimate debasement of traditional Chinese herbal medicine occurs when chemists try to find "active principles" in Chinese herbal formulas, and pull from these complex mixtures a single extracted drug. Chinese herbalists laugh at these attempts, but it is a sorrowful laugh, for the Western approach appears to be winning. The sophisticated tradition of Chinese herbology is rapidly degenerating into a mere resource for exploitation.

I sincerely hope this fate may be avoided; that, through the work of Dr. Chan and others, the artfulness of Oriental herbology may survive and flourish.

How to Use Chinese Herbology

To use Chinese herbs properly, I advise against purchasing them from health food stores or through pyramid marketing schemes. Oriental herbology is too sophisticated an art to be practiced as a form of self-treatment. A trained herbalist is essential.

In my experience the best Chinese herbalists are usually associated with acupuncture schools. Also, many traditional Oriental herb stores have herbalists on staff who know what they are doing. However, they sometimes do not speak English well.

Most acupuncturists also prescribe Chinese herbs, but not all have been adequately trained in the art of herbology. Insist on whole-person formulas rather than symptomatic treatments. I also recommend checking the number of hours of herbal training the acupuncturist has undertaken. Five hundred hours is probably the minimum necessary for competency.

Efficacy of Chinese Herbal Treatment

There have not been enough good studies performed on the effectiveness of traditional Chinese herbal formulas to make any objective statement about their general efficacy. Because of its individualized nature, proper Chinese herbal treatment is almost as difficult to study as acupuncture. Nonetheless, good research is being performed, especially in Japan, and in a number of years it should be possible to make more definitive statements.

Until that time, clinical experience is the only guide. Chinese herbology in the hands of a competent practitioner is in my judgment far more potent and effective than Western herbology. In many cases it rivals or exceeds the effectiveness of drugs.

Safety of Chinese Herbs

Like Western herbs, many Chinese herbs are used in cooking. They are imported as foods and are considered safe on a presumptive basis. However, Chinese herbal practitioners also use herbs that are not used in cooking, herbs that may be potentially toxic. Their safety has not been fully evaluated scientifically. But because they have been used for so many centuries, safe dosages have long ago been determined.

Nonetheless, Chinese herbology is traditionally recognized as being more dangerous than acupuncture. This is not because of fears of toxicity, but simply out of respect for the power of Oriental herbal medicine. Improperly performed acupuncture will seldom do more than cause a brief flare-up of pain. But an incorrectly chosen herbal combination is supposed to be able to make patients sicker.

A further consideration is the possibility that there may be long-delayed dangers of Chinese herbs, or consequences that occur only rarely. Such problems might reasonably be expected to have escaped the scrutiny of generations of herbalists. It is next to impossible to discover rare or delayed side effects without national registries and systematic surveys, such as exist for drugs. Therefore, it is possible that some Chinese herbs may cause harmful effects that have never been identified.

Similarly, it is generally not known whether a given Chinese herb interacts adversely with drugs. The subject simply has not been studied satisfactorily.

Finally, Chinese herbs present a unique problem regarding pesticides and other contaminants. Because these herbs are grown in the Third World, they may have been treated with pesticides or other chemicals that are banned in the United States. Residues may linger in herbal products, causing unexpected problems. Some highly allergic people have bad reactions to Chinese herbs, reactions that may be caused by these artificial additives.

Eventually, Chinese herbs will be grown in the West under more wholesome conditions. This is part of the larger process of adapting Asian medical insights to the modern world, a task that is both fraught with difficulties and rich in opportunities.

CHAPTER 7

Bodywork:
The Real Physical Therapy

Under the heading "bodywork" I include all those crafts of healing that involve hands-on skills of touch, massage, and movement. Such methods do not depend primarily on intellectual skills. Rather, these silent, persevering endeavors of the hands and fingers require tactile gifts, a high level of body awareness, and extensive practice.

The four main categories of bodywork are massage (and its variations), chiropractic, movement therapy, and osteopathy. Each of these has its uses, abuses, and limitations, and its higher and lower forms.

Physical therapy is actually a form of bodywork. Because it is part of conventional medicine, however, physical therapists feel a need to quantify and define their work. They memorize muscle attachments and hunger after computerized strain gauges. Too much influenced by the medical model, they often rely on cognitive skills rather than trusting their hands to guide them.

In contrast, the best bodyworkers are primarily "right-brained." They think with their fingers; they know what they know by feel and by touch. I have found some of the deepest practitioners of the arts of healing among bodyworkers.

Bodywork fulfills many of the ideals of alternative medicine. It is safe, natural, and noninterventive. Furthermore, the higher forms of bodywork can heal at a deep level and may even prevent future injuries.

Ellen Karstein's story demonstrates the importance of the bodywork arts in the treatment of pain. Her first words to me were familiar: "I have tried everything and none of it has helped me." This forty-three-year-old mother of two told me of her auto accident four years earlier. Her medical doctor had prescribed anti-inflammatory medications and muscle relaxants and suggested she wear a cervical collar. One month later, Mrs. Karstein still hurt. The doctor then sent her for X rays, an MRI (magnetic resonance imaging exam), and two nerve conduction studies. They showed nothing. Next, he prescribed an antidepressant and referred her for twenty sessions with a physical therapist. Six months later, Ellen's pain was no better.

With little hope in her voice, she asked me whether there was any chance alternative medicine could help control her pain. I assured her that it was quite likely, and then surprised her by saying that she had scarcely exhausted her options. "To tell you the truth," I said, "you haven't even begun to try the methods that might really help you."

She was incredulous. "I've been going to doctors two or three times a week for years."

"Yes, but nothing you have tried up to this point offered much chance of success. To have tried conventional treatment is practically not to have tried any treatment at all."

I recommended chiropractic and acupuncture, and within six months her pain was permanently cured. I hadn't been exaggerating. Her problem was not so difficult; it was just that nothing she had tried had any chance of succeeding.

Muscle relaxants and antidepressants almost never relieve neck pain satisfactorily and, if they do, the effect is ordinarily short-lived. After a month or so, they stop working. Anti-inflammatory medications also provide only a little relief, and they carry real risk of stomach ulcers and other serious problems.

Nerve conduction studies, MRIs, and X rays are tests, not treatments. They do not cure anything in themselves. Their only use is to determine whether there is a serious underlying problem, such as a fracture, a ruptured disk, or a tumor. When these studies come out negative, as they usually do, a doctor can offer no more than a referral to physical therapy.

Unfortunately, ordinary physical therapy (PT) for neck pain is a bit of a sham. Many physical therapists have admitted this to me, as did the administrator of a major health maintenance organization. "Our own internal studies," he said, "show that when it comes to chronic neck, back, and shoulder pain, physical therapy does not work any better than doing nothing at all. To be consistent with our own guidelines, we should stop sending many of our patients for PT. Unfortunately, doctors and patients demand it. Personally, I think standard physical therapy for neck pain is nothing more than an expensive placebo."

Physical therapy can be very useful in other circumstances. Following a stroke or a spinal injury, for example, physical therapists can provide invaluable rehabilitation services. But the typical treatment modalities for neck pain—hot and cold packs, ultrasound, diathermy, and simplistic exercises—seldom provide more than temporary relief. (Some physical therapists have supplemented their basic skills with healing arts such as muscle energy manipulation or myofascial release, or use sophisticated exercise systems like Med-x or Pilates. These practitioners can be quite effective.)

When physical therapy fails, medical doctors have few options. Most are reluctant to recommend surgery for neck pain, because the outcome can easily be worse than the original problem. They may refer patients to chronic pain centers. Unfortunately, many of the treatments provided by pain clinics (such as epidural steroid injections) are nearly ineffective.

In other words, the whole range of medical options for chronic neck or back pain amounts to little more than a hope that time will provide a cure. Like the emperor's new clothes, medical treatment for these conditions does not really exist.

In my opinion, a person with neck or back pain should use conventional medicine only to rule out potentially dangerous possibilities. For treatment, the patient should look to alternative medicine, especially to acupuncture and the various bodywork arts.

Because it requires many sessions and is labor-intensive, bodywork is relatively expensive. And it may fail. While it is often extremely helpful, bodywork is no magic panacea. Sometimes the technique used by the bodyworker is insufficient. "Plain vanilla" massage, for example, seldom produces more than temporary relief. Even if the technique is sophisticated, the bodyworker must possess a high level of skill to make it work. Therefore, a mediocre Rolfer may not be able to cure a single case of chronic neck pain, although Rolfing itself is a wonderful technique.

At times the lifestyle of the patient blocks success. I remember a woman whose hip pain seemed incurable. Only after three months of treatment did she happen to mention that she went skydiving almost every weekend! Extreme life stress or physically injurious working conditions may also stand in the way of recovery.

In some cases, pain simply may be too advanced or too difficult for anyone to treat. This is particularly the case when a patient has already had neck or back surgery.

Finally, there are many mysterious situations where a condition that does not seem difficult proves impossible to cure. I have no explanation for these all-too-common occurrences other than to say that healing itself remains a mystery.

In the following pages, I describe the most important branches of bodywork.

MASSAGE

The simplest form of bodywork and the most widely available is basic therapeutic massage. Generic massage includes elements of the traditional Swedish method: primarily stroking, kneading, and rubbing of the superficial muscles. These are usually combined with the light, soothing massage techniques developed in the 1960s at the Esalen Institute in Big Sur, California. Another common form of massage is the "hurts good and feels great when it's over" style known as deep-tissue work.

Massage of this type can reduce stress and relieve the pain of aching muscles. Many people find that regular massage sessions increase their sense of vitality and overall well-being. Further claims have been made that massage can speed recovery from illnesses, help injured tissues heal, and release buried emotional traumas.

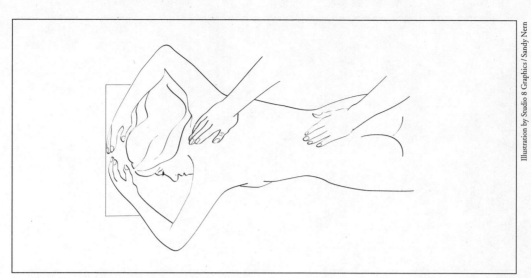

Illustration by Studio 8 Graphics / Sandy Nern

Figure 7.1 Massage can relieve stress and aching muscles.

While generic massage is adequate for mild discomfort, it is not particularly effective as a treatment for more severe chronic pain. Its effects seldom last for more than a day or two. Ordinarily, more advanced techniques are necessary to produce long-lasting results. (The only exception to this rule occurs when the massage therapist happens to possess extraordinary natural gifts. Technique is one thing, talent quite another.)

Neuromuscular therapy, muscle energy manipulation, myofascial release, and Rolfing are variations on the theme of massage that go several steps beyond the basic art. In some cases these methods can make a significant contribution to recovery from chronic pain.

Neuromuscular Therapy

Several forms of neuromuscular work are available. Perhaps the most famous of these is the St. John method. These techniques focus on specific muscles, applying finger pressure not only to the large "muscle bellies," but also to the tendinous attachments at each end of a muscle. Neuromuscular therapy requires detailed anatomical knowledge and study of the pathways by which pain spreads through the body.

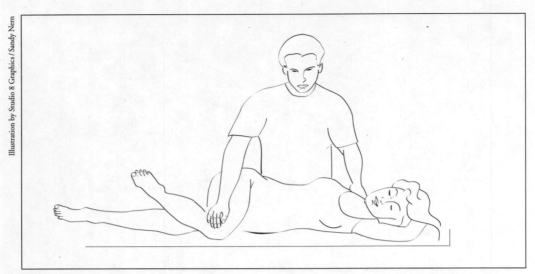

Illustration by Studio 8 Graphics / Sandy Nern

Figure 7.2 Muscle energy manipulation. One position involves pushing the patient's shoulder down while simultaneously pushing down the opposite knee.

Methods of this type can be useful in the treatment of problems such as rotator cuff tear, tendinitis, thoracic outlet syndrome, and torticollis. Neuromuscular therapy is less likely to be effective for problems involving large complexes of muscles, such as neck and back pain.

Muscle Energy Manipulation

This method originated in osteopathy, but it is widely used today by massage therapists and unconventional physical therapists. It involves having the patient push against resistance applied by the therapist. One form of the work involves sophisticated techniques for working with the deep muscles of the pelvis in order to stabilize and correct faulty structure. This particular procedure can be quite useful in the treatment of back pain. In general, muscle energy manipulation is a moderately effective technique for chronic pain of muscular origin. I sometimes recommend it when more acute-care methods such as chiropractic have failed.

Myofascial Release

This technique also originated in osteopathy. It involves fairly intense manipulation of the fascia, the sheathing tissues that coat all the muscles of the body. Myofascial release is particularly effective for plantar fasciitis, frozen shoulder, carpal tunnel syndrome, fibromyalgia, myofascial pain syndrome, tendinitis, and thoracic outlet syndrome, but it can also be used for many other chronic muscular pain syndromes. However, some patients find it too painful.

Rolfing

Rolfing is probably the most sophisticated of the massage-related techniques. It was founded in the 1950s by a biochemist and genius of the hand, Ida Rolfe. The Rolfing theory of structural integration is based on two principles: the power of gravity and the importance of the fascia.

The power of gravity. Ida Rolfe took as her starting point the obvious fact that our bodies are engaged in a constant interaction with the force of gravity. Next, she realized that because of gravity an injury to one part of the body affects the whole. To understand her insight, consider the effects of a back injury on a previously healthy person.

When uninjured, a person walks upright, in line with the pull of gravity. This is the position in which the body is best able to deal with the eternal downward pull. But after an injury, pain may force a person to walk slightly bent forward. This small alteration of normal posture changes the effect of gravity's pull on the entire body. Operating on a bent spine, gravity pulls forward as well as straight down. Therefore the muscles of the lower back must pull backward to stop the person from toppling forward. The hamstrings and other leg muscles necessarily join in the struggle to keep the body stable in its new position, and the various muscles of the neck and shoulder girdle come into play to keep the head erect.

Such a reorganization of muscular function produces discomfort and pain. Thus, from a single injury the whole musculoskeletal system suffers. As in a building that has begun to sag, the force of gravity alters the normal stress patterns

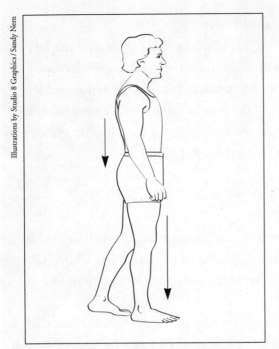

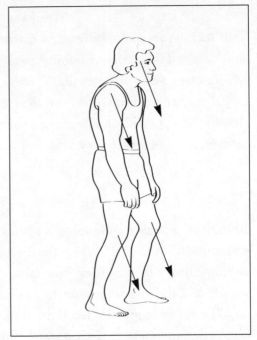

Figure 7.3 A person walking in line with the downward pull of gravity.

Figure 7.4 Poor posture causes gravity to pull forward as well as downward.

throughout the entire structure. If nothing is done to set such a building or body right again, it may collapse. It must be pulled "back into true."

The Importance of the Fascia. Rolfe next asked herself why the body doesn't simply realign itself when the original injury heals. Unlike a house, the human body possesses a self-restoring power. It ought to be able to reestablish normal posture.

In her search for an explanation, Rolfe looked at the tough, semitransparent fascial tissues that surround all the muscles of the body. Rolfe's observations led her to conclude that these tissues are the real culprit. She believed that when an injury lasts for a while, the fascia become stretched, distorted, and moved out of proper position. Even when the original injury is resolved, these distorted fascial tissues can influence the muscles to remain out of proper alignment.

Once she understood this, Rolfe developed a technique for manipulating the fascia back into proper alignment. This is what has become known as the Rolfe Method of Structural Integration, or Rolfing for short.

Ten Sessions. Rolfing employs a series of ten sessions to systematically restore proper position to the fascial tissues. Like myofascial release, the work can be rather intense, but in recent years Rolfers have tended to modify their method to produce less pain. Each session focuses on certain areas of the body, so that by the end the entire structure has been manipulated. The result is meant to be a body that is properly aligned in space, floating upright in the sea of gravity. This goal is similar to that espoused by chiropractic, but sought through the soft tissues rather than the bones.

Rolfing can produce remarkable improvements in posture. It also can be quite helpful for pain syndromes involving many muscle groups, such as chronic neck and back pain. However, in my experience, Rolfing does not successfully relieve chronic pain as often as its sophisticated theory would seem to promise. Chiropractic, acupuncture, neuromuscular therapy, muscle energy work, myofascial release, and the Feldenkrais method (described later) seem to produce good results more reliably. I ordinarily recommend these other techniques first and try Rolfing only if the outcome is still unsatisfactory. An indication of the order in which to apply these methods for specific problems may be found in section V.

Oriental Forms of Massage

Another sophisticated form of massage therapy is Shiatsu, or acupressure. This is actually a branch of Oriental medicine, and it requires considerable practice and sensitivity to perform effectively. In Japan the profession is mostly reserved for the blind, who alone are considered capable of the intense tactile concentration the technique requires for success. Skillful practitioners are supposed to be able to reproduce many of the results of acupuncture without using needles. However, few Western practitioners are sufficiently competent in Shiatsu to produce results other than temporary relief from pain.

Other oriental bodywork techniques practiced in the United States include Jinshin Jyutsu, Sotai, "inner aikido," and Jinshin Do. All these systems share many of the principles of acupuncture and Oriental medicine.

Emotion-Release Massage

Many massage therapists have noticed that massage can provoke surprisingly specific emotional responses. For example, the manipulation of a shoulder or arm may provoke cathartic emotional experiences related in some way to that part of the body. These "body memories" may include intense fits of anger or panic, loud sobbing, or vivid flashbacks to events of the past.

Certain forms of massage therapy aim deliberately at producing emotional releases. These include SOMA, the Rosen method, and some of John Upledger's techniques. Their most significant use is in the emotional rather than the physical arena, although they can sometimes relieve chronic pain as well.

Some practitioners of these methods are highly skillful. However, not everyone who practices emotion-release massage is adequately trained to deal with the emotional reactions that occur. It is always a good idea to involve a trained psychotherapist as well when using these methods.

A step further in this direction are forms of psychotherapy that use physical contact as a tool. Some of these body-oriented psychotherapy techniques are addressed in chapter 8.

CHIROPRACTIC

Because I advertise myself as an alternative doctor, people often come to me for advice when conventional medicine fails them. I view it as my job to sort through the various possibilities and suggest those alternatives most likely to succeed. This is what Harvey Larsen had in mind when he consulted me regarding his right-sided abdominal and groin pain. When he heard my suggestion, however, he wondered whether he could trust me.

Harvey was a forty-five-year-old accountant who came to my Olympia, Washington, office during September 1993. While blacktopping his driveway, Harvey felt a sudden tearing sensation in his groin. He spent an uncomfortable night and visited his doctor in the morning. The family physician diagnosed an inflamed prostate.

"An inflamed prostate?" I interrupted in surprise. "How is that connected to working on your driveway?"

"I wondered about that too," Harvey replied, then went on with his story. I listened in growing amazement. Harvey had taken three courses of antibiotics, visited four specialists, and undergone a biopsy, a laparoscopy, and numerous diagnostic tests. None of the doctors seemed to make any connection between Harvey's pain and the physical effort of blacktopping a driveway. What a wild goose chase! Lacking one essential piece of information, they missed the obvious diagnosis.

Harvey's remarkable journey through the world of medicine finally led to my office. He was terribly frustrated. If anything, his pain was now worse than it had been at the beginning. Harvey asked me whether alternative medicine could help him. I paused before answering, still marveling at his story.

"Mr. Larsen," I finally said, "I'm sorry you went through all those medical procedures. I'm afraid that they were a bit irrelevant. It seems to me that your prostate problem was completely unrelated to your pain. Working on your driveway wouldn't cause you to get a sudden prostate infection. You might have had prostatitis for years. It was a red herring. What you need now is the same as what you needed in the beginning. You need to see a chiropractor."

His look of hopeful anticipation evaporated into an expression of disgust. Shaking his head emphatically, Harvey explained, "I don't trust chiropractors. I would *never, never* go to a chiropractor."

Because so many people distrust chiropractors, his vehement reaction did not surprise me. Chiropractic is in the peculiar position of being simultaneously the most successful alternative health care profession and perhaps the least respected. A large segment of the population puts chiropractors in the same class as used-car salesmen.

To some extent chiropractic has earned this reputation through its own practices. This is unfortunate, as chiropractic manipulation is an important treatment option. For decades, legitimate scientific research validating the worth of chiropractic treatment has been accumulating. In 1994 a government agency finally made it official: spinal manipulation works! The Agency for Health Care Policy and Research (AHCPR, a branch of the federal Health and Human Services

Department) issued guidelines recommending spinal manipulation as a first-line treatment for acute low-back pain. Evaluations of chiropractic treatment for other common pain conditions are forthcoming.

Such recognition is long overdue. I consider chiropractic the treatment of choice for many musculoskeletal pain problems. In cases of neck and back pain, spinal manipulation is faster (on average) than acupuncture, more effective than massage therapy, and far more useful than conventional medicine. Painful joints and sore muscles frequently respond to chiropractic as well. I recommend that anyone injured in an automobile accident should see a good D.C. (doctor of chiropractic) within the first week.

Harvey needed to see a chiropractor because he had strained his psoas muscle while blacktopping. Any chiropractor would have made the diagnosis at once. In the language of the profession, Harvey suffered from the common problem known as psoas spasm.

Many people are not aware of their psoas muscle. Traveling by a hidden route deep inside the pelvis, it connects the lower spine to the inside of the leg. There is no way to directly palpate or touch this muscle. Prolonged squatting is one activity that can injure the psoas. Because it produces lower abdominal and groin pain, psoas spasm is commonly confused with pelvic inflammatory disease, inguinal hernia, ovarian cyst, prostatitis, and various digestive disorders.

Most medical doctors have never heard of psoas spasm. I never encountered the phrase while I was in medical school. Even if a doctor were able to diagnose this problem, he or she would have little to offer. Conventional medicine lacks adequate tools for treating muscle spasms generally. This is the real reason Harvey's doctors ignored the obvious muscular cause of his pain and instead investigated his prostate gland: it is human nature to pay most attention to problems one knows how to confront. Medical doctors have many tools to address prostate infections, and none for psoas spasms. Therefore, they gave Harvey antibiotics.

In contrast, psoas and other muscle spasms are basic subjects in the chiropractic curriculum. All chiropractic students learn to diagnose and treat these problems. I was quite confident that a few sessions with a good D.C. would relieve Harvey's discomfort. However, I couldn't get him to go. Only after I delivered the entire contents of this chapter in spoken form would he consent to take my suggestion. As I expected, my colleague Dr. David Chedre quickly relieved his pain.

Many people are in Harvey's position. They suffer from a condition chiropractic can cure, but chiropractic's poor image makes them afraid to try. Their medical doctors do nothing to change their minds. Therefore, they avoid the one treatment that is most appropriate.

How Does Chiropractic Manipulation Work?

As for acupuncture, the honest answer to this question is, "No one really knows." For years chiropractors have claimed that spinal manipulation "corrects vertebral subluxations," or "out-of-place" vertebrae, by putting them back in place. The traditional chiropractic X rays are supposed to identify which vertebrae need to be manipulated, and the satisfying cracking noises heard during a session are supposed to be the sounds of bone shifting position.

However, there is little evidence that spinal manipulation immediately changes the position of any vertebrae. (Visible improvements actually can occur over a period of many months of treatment.) Postsession X ray films typically look the same as presession films. In other words, although they undoubtedly relieve pain, chiropractic "adjustments" may not actually adjust anything. The famous chiropractic sounds may be no different than the gas bubble noises that are heard when knuckles "crack."

A group of revisionist chiropractors have begun to abandon the old notion of subluxations and adjustment. According to them, the true effect of chiropractic manipulation is to loosen stuck spots in the spine and adjacent muscles. These they call "spinal fixations." Although this explanation has yet to be proved correct, the available studies seem to indicate that it is closer to the truth than the "adjusting spinal subluxations" explanation.

Fortunately, as with all crafts, an exact explanation of how spinal manipulation works doesn't really matter. Numerous good studies and the experience of millions of patients have shown that, however it actually functions, spinal manipulation can bring relief from pain.

How Well Does Chiropractic Work?

This question is difficult to answer precisely. Like every healing art, chiropractic lacks a comprehensive research foundation. Hands-on techniques like chiropractic are difficult if not impossible to work into double-blind protocols. Furthermore, unlike conventional medicine, chiropractic did not originate as a branch of Western science. Until recently, its practitioners have not made rigorous research a high priority. Finally, as a practical matter it is difficult to obtain funding for chiropractic research. There is no deep-pocket equivalent of pharmaceutical companies to cough up the cash, and university investigators with access to grant money tend to turn their attention to higher-tech subjects.

Nonetheless, good chiropractic research does exist. I have already mentioned the federal AHCPR report on back pain. This was actually a review of studies. The authors looked at all the available literature and concluded that spinal manipulation was one of the best (and best documented) treatments available for recent-onset back pain.

Other substantive research has demonstrated that chiropractic can be useful and cost-effective in the treatment of headaches and neck pain. Not all of these studies were well-designed, but taken together they form a body of strong evidence in favor of spinal manipulation as a treatment for a variety of conditions.

This is significant in itself and provides grounds for funding of future research. However, the total body of available solid information is insufficient to fully guide treatment in real-life situations. For example, not enough research has been performed to evaluate such important questions as: Does chiropractic work for chronic back and neck pain as well as it does for acute injury? Are there subtypes of neck and back pain that respond best to treatment? How many chiropractic treatments should be sufficient, on average, for each type of problem? Does regular chiropractic prevent future exacerbations of pain? Does it produce any other beneficial effects?

Pending future data, the answers to these questions can only be given roughly, on the grounds of clinical impression. I draw the following conclusions from my experience of working closely with numerous excellent chiropractors, referring patients to them, and discussing with them what they have observed.

In my opinion, chiropractic is the first treatment to try for neck or back pain. For these problems, it is much more powerful than massage and often provides quicker relief than any other alternative option. Nothing in conventional medicine rivals it. (Indeed, conventional medicine is almost useless for neck and back pain.) Chiropractic is most effective for pain of less than three months' duration, but it often helps chronic conditions as well.

Other conditions for which chiropractic is frequently helpful include muscle spasms (including internal muscles like the diaphragm and psoas), shoulder pain, knee pain, and headaches. Pain in other joints sometimes responds to chiropractic too, but less often. Finally, spinal manipulation can occasionally shift a breech presentation in pregnancy.

How Is Chiropractic Best Used?

Generally, it is better to get chiropractic treatment early rather than late. For example, many patients who suffer periodic attacks of neck or back pain observe that their spasms are preceded by weeks or months of increasing tension. A few sessions of chiropractic manipulation in the early stages of the buildup will often suffice to avert the onset of a spasm. But if treatment is not begun until after severe neck pain has developed, it may take many more chiropractic treatments to restore comfort.

For this reason, I always recommend visiting a good chiropractor immediately after an auto accident. Not only does spinal manipulation relieve pain in the short term, in my clinical experience early chiropractic care can sometimes prevent a drawn-out recovery process. A condition may become complicated and hard to treat after many months have elapsed without treatment.

I advise trying no more than ten sessions of chiropractic initially. If there is partial relief, it is worthwhile trying another ten. But if there is no relief at all after ten sessions, further care with that chiropractic physician probably will not help.

Like acupuncture, chiropractic is not a commodity. There are nearly two hundred distinct chiropractic methods and a wide range of competence among physicians. Therefore, sometimes one chiropractor can succeed where another fails.

Treatment on an occasional or as-needed basis can be appropriate for recurrent conditions. But I strongly advise against continuing weekly or biweekly chiropractic treatment for months or years if it isn't working. Why keep trying chiropractic when there are so many other good options available? If chiropractic fails, I suggest switching to acupuncture or, even better, combining the two. As I mentioned earlier, acupuncture and chiropractic support one another. One chiropractic adjustment combined with one acupuncture treatment is usually better than two sessions of either method alone.

For difficult chronic pain problems that do not respond to acupuncture or chiropractic, I often recommend one of the sophisticated variants of massage, or Feldenkrais therapy (described later in this chapter). Feldenkrais is particularly useful for problems that respond to treatment briefly but then return. For example, many individuals find that chiropractic relieves back pain for a day or a week, but their backs predictably "go out" again soon. Feldenkrais can retrain the body so that it becomes more stable and resilient, reducing the incidence of these reinjuries. Rolfing can sometimes produce similarly good results.

Is Chiropractic Good for Other Problems Besides Pain?

In my opinion, chiropractic's utility is entirely limited to the treatment of pain. Many chiropractors will disagree. They still hold to the older view that spinal manipulation can cure many diseases.

This idea dates back to the turn of the century. Daniel Palmer, the founder of chiropractic, believed he had discovered in spinal manipulation the cause and cure of nearly all diseases. He imagined that every illness stemmed from vertebral subluxations restricting nerve outflows. It was a tidy theory, doing away with all medicine and surgery in a single sweep. Unfortunately, spinal manipulation has not proved to be a useful solution for many health problems besides pain.

The public seems to understand this. Most people who visit chiropractors do so for treatment of musculoskeletal pain alone. But the profession seems unable to let go entirely of its past grand claims. Too many chiropractors still talk about curing internal illnesses through manipulation. They tell wonderful anecdotes of chiropractic curing deafness, asthma, and even cancer.

No doubt some of these tales are true. It is a phenomenon seen throughout alternative medicine: serious problems are occasionally cured by methods that do not succeed very often. Royal jelly and spirulina juice can boast as many miracle cures as chiropractic. However, none of these healing substances produces miracles regularly. The same may be said of chiropractic.

Healing is mysterious. While I do not pretend to be able to explain how royal jelly and chiropractic can occasionally cure serious internal illnesses, I know by experience that such events are rare. In real life, chiropractic often helps painful backs but hardly ever cures bladder infections, diabetes, or even a common cold, as most chiropractors will admit.

Some advocates claim that regular chiropractic care can keep the body healthy. While such statements are easy to make, they are not easy to show. Personally, I think that it is a healthy lifestyle that most effectively prevents disease. What any physician can contribute beyond this is much less significant.

Should Chiropractors
Be Used as Primary Care Physicians?

Chiropractic is definitely a useful form of bodywork. Furthermore, most chiropractors are fully capable of managing the treatment of pain, including making referrals when necessary. But some chiropractors believe themselves to be all-round primary care doctors as well.

While chiropractic education does provide considerable book learning on medical subjects, there is simply no comparison between a family practitioner's and a chiropractor's clinical training in general medicine. Chiropractic students receive a relatively minuscule amount of hands-on experience with patients suffering from actual diseases. Most of their clinical time is spent on the conditions for which patients ordinarily seek chiropractic care, mainly neck and back pain. By contrast, a family practice resident is up to the elbows in medical diseases sixty hours a week for several years of training.

Without practical experience, the information does not come alive. Chiropractors have never seen instances of half the subjects they've read about; therefore, their knowledge is all theory. Furthermore, no matter how good their education, after graduation chiropractors spend most of their time practicing spinal manipulation. Meanwhile, conventional doctors are busy putting into practice everything they've learned, and learning more.

My friend Dr. Chedre is acutely aware of his limitations, but some of his colleagues compound inexperience with overconfidence. These are the D.C.s who commit the sins of misdiagnosis and mistreatment for which chiropractic is often criticized. They simply do not know how much they do not know.

I wish chiropractors would let go of their "physician wanna-be" attitudes and simply take pride in their unique skill at treating pain. To me, being an excellent bodyworker and a pain specialist is honor enough. This is the path taken by those chiropractors whom I most respect.

Chiropractors Who Sell Supplements

In many states chiropractors function as de facto naturopaths, selling a wide variety of herbs and supplements. Some of these practitioners are well-trained in modern naturopathy and provide an adequate service along the lines described in chapter 4. Others, however, tend to follow fads more closely than basic science, and indulge in many of the least savory forms of naturopathic treatment.

Problems with Chiropractic

Chiropractors often complain that their profession is not taken seriously. While it is true that the medical profession has unfairly maligned chiropractic for decades, chiropractic has cooperated by making itself a vulnerable target for those attacks. I am a strong supporter of the technique of chiropractic manipulation, but I feel that the profession of chiropractic has some serious problems. These may be grouped into two categories: excessive commercialism and chronically low standards of truth.

Commercialism. Chiropractic as a whole seems to tolerate an astonishing level of blatant commercialism. Too many chiropractors behave more like retail salesmen than responsible health care providers.

All the chiropractors whom I have come to respect have confessed they feel embarassed by the actions of many of their colleagues. Dr. Chedre has told me that the atmosphere of his chiropractic college was more reminiscent of a motivational sales course than a serious study. Guest speakers came to brag of their two-million-dollar-a-year practices and explained, with a straight face, that the higher their incomes, the more patients they know they helped.

Chiropractic itself is ideally suited for making money on an industrial scale. If performed cynically, the techniques of spinal manipulation can yield a satisfying series of cracks in under a minute. This allows for tremendous patient volume. Many chiropractors offer a free spinal exam as a kind of loss leader. Inevitably, patients are found to have many subluxations. They are told they need a full course of X rays and frequent treatments extending far into the future. The joke goes: "How many chiropractors does it take to change a light bulb?" Answer: "Just one, but he has to change it three times a week for twenty years!"

Conventional medicine has its obvious and less-obvious commercial aspects too, but they are not so blatant. If chiropractic wishes to improve its social standing as a respectable profession, it must adopt a less grasping stance.

Low Standards of Truth. Beyond casual commercialism, chiropractic also damages its reputation by indulging in extremely incautious statements. For example, many chiropractors have a chart on the wall that shows how vertebral misalignment, unless corrected by chiropractic adjustment, inevitably progresses into spinal arthritis. Most people have come to expect that when professionals make statements like these, they are speaking out of reliable knowledge. However, such is not the case with chiropractic. This particular claim has been promulgated for a hundred years without any solid evidence to support it. To my knowledge, no randomized longitudinal studies have ever compared patients who receive adjustments with those who do not. Therefore, it is impossible to know whether regular adjustment prevents spinal arthritis. The idea is simply a self-serving one. A reputable profession should not make such unsupported statements.

Because of these serious problems with the profession, I feel that I have to choose carefully before recommending a chiropractor to my patients. Nonetheless, I regularly recommend chiropractic. I believe it to be an important and useful treatment for nearly all conditions of chronic pain.

Dangers of Chiropractic Spinal Manipulation

Some people fear that spinal manipulation can cause fractures, strokes, and other major injuries. I have never encountered such a case myself, and available statistics show that these complications are rare to nonexistent. It is true that chiropractic can cause temporary exacerbation of pain. However, only those who have severe osteoporosis, spinal fracture, or other unusual pathology need fear serious adverse consequences from chiropractic treatment.

The most fundamental problem of chiropractic is one it shares with every other system of healing: chiropractic may not work, yet chiropractors may be reluctant to admit the fact. They may keep treating a patient for years when it would have been better to admit defeat and suggest acupuncture or a different form of bodywork.

Will Insurance Pay for Chiropractic?

Chiropractic is reimbursed by insurance much more reliably than any other form of alternative medicine. Frequently, however, there are limits to the total number of visits allowed. This is actually quite reasonable, as a chiropractic treatment is usually a pleasant experience. Without such limits, insurance companies could be liable for unlimited expenses.

How to Pick a Chiropractor

As in all healing crafts, choosing a good chiropractor is extremely important. A huge range exists between the best and the worst. In my personal estimation (without the benefit of any statistical evidence) about 30 percent of all chiropractors are not worth seeing for reasons of excessive commercialism. Another 50 percent avoid this tendency, but their bodywork skills are too limited to offer a great deal of help. Only about 20 percent are truly skilled bodyworkers and take the time to apply their skills properly.

Bad chiropractors will probably not cause injury, but they will deplete your checking account. A moderately skilled D.C. can offer some relief, but for the best results it is essential to seek excellence.

Of course, chiropractors do not publicly rank themselves as "money hungry" or "minimally skilled." Referral services can't legitimately make these distinctions either. Here, as with all healing arts, there is no substitute for seasoned discrimination. For this reason, I will devote the remaining pages of this subsection to the important task of choosing a chiropractor.

A technique I use to locate superior chiropractors in a new area is to interview individuals who have had long experience with chiropractic care. Through visiting many chiropractors over the years, they have usually developed a reliable basis from which to compare. Conversely, patients who love their chiropractor but have never seen any other practitioner are not trustworthy referral sources. They may have simply "swallowed the line" of a good salesman. I always find that the recommendations given by experienced patients in a given area converge on two or three local D.C.s.

Those chiropractors with the biggest buildings, the most advertisements, and the greatest political clout are often the worst at actual treatment. Such practitioners may be more gifted at the glib arts of marketing than at the diligent persistence required to actualize a healing craft.

The best chiropractors possess the following characteristics: Although they may sell a few supplements or espouse a few unusual theories, they are essentially bodyworkers at heart. They spend at least twenty minutes with each patient in direct hands-on work. They take X rays only rarely and avoid massage machines and other gadgets. Prior to spinal manipulation, they perform trigger-point release or some other soft-tissue technique.

These sincere healers make no promises and know when to stop. Their offices and advertisements are small, their practices moderate in size, and they use no clever practice management schemes. Instead, they hope to succeed through skill and hard work. They often ask for payment in cash, being more adept at body-work than at filling out insurance forms.

To help the reader recognize these patterns of practice, I will conclude this chapter by profiling some actual chiropractors (under assumed names). It is my hope that these portraits will aid the reader in making a discriminating selection.

Profile of a "Rack-'em, Stack-'em, and Crack-'em" Chiropractor. Shortly after I opened a holistic practice in a large Midwestern town, Dr. Silver invited me to visit his office. Ornate Grecian pillars framed the entrance to his solid brick clinic. Inside, the spacious waiting room was beautifully decorated with Oriental rugs. A white board listed "the best referring patients," with red stars next to the top ten.

Dr. Silver beamed at me when I entered his office. After the introductions were over, he decided to let me in on the secrets of his success. "It all starts with the waiting room," he explained. "If patients see a full waiting room, they know you must be busy. If you're busy, you must be good. My office manager schedules appointments in such a way as to keep the waiting room full at all times. That's very important."

"Now, let me tell you how we treat our patients. After they've had their X rays, we send them to the 'spinalator.' It's a mechanical massage table. Ten minutes on that, and we can bill a code for massage. The machines are all paid off, so it's pure profit. And, it makes them feel great."

He smiled broadly before continuing. "Next, my patients go to the hot-and-cold room. We have infrared lamps, cold packs, the works. Whatever their policy pays for, they get. So far, I've billed fifty dollars or more, and I haven't even seen the patient yet. Quite a system, eh? Finally, I step in, give them some personal bonding, and make 'em crack from stem to stern. They like it good and loud.

"I'm a believer in customer service, you know. I never make them pay their copayment. I never even show them the total bill. It goes straight to the insurance company." He flashed a conspiratorial grin. "No reason to make them tense up as they walk out the door." (Routinely ignoring copayments is illegal, although it is a common practice.)

"I never forget to send them cards on their birthday," Dr. Silver continued. "It helps them realize that I care. Also, I reward them for referrals by putting their names on the board. They eat it up. They feel like they're part of the family. Of course, I don't hesitate to advertise. You have to spend money to make money. My advertising budget is five thousand dollars a month."

Dr. Silver paused and gave me a concerned look. "I hope you understand that this isn't materialistic. It's about service to humanity. If you make more money, it means you're helping more people. I feel really good about what I'm doing."

I believe he did. Dr. Silver's conception of his mission in life could be described as a bit shallow. Needless to say, I didn't refer any patients his way. Not that he needed my referrals—he saw five hundred patients each week, a number it takes me more than three months to reach. I have heard of chiropractors who see twice as many.

Profile of an Excellent Chiropractor. Dr. David Chedre is the kind of chiropractor I send my patients to. He works out of a small office, with only one secretary, and uses no marketing techniques other than the quality of his work. He never takes X rays himself, but if he feels that an X ray would be useful, he sends his patients to a nearby medical radiology laboratory.

Unlike Dr. Silver, Dr. Chedre can seldom finish a session in less than twenty minutes. His method is slow and painstaking and, obviously, no way to get rich. But it is an excellent way to help patients feel better.

Dr. Chedre spends at least ten minutes working with the muscles and soft tissues before he "cracks" the spine. With considerable skill, he uses methods drawn from a wide variety of bodywork arts, including Japanese physical therapy, myofascial release, and muscle energy work. His fingers are skillful and work with an intelligence of their own. In his hands, chiropractic is a refined and supple instrument for healing, a truly sophisticated form of bodywork.

"That's what I am, a bodyworker," Chedre says smiling. "And I'm proud of it."

He also teaches exercise that patients can do at home and provides guidance on proper movement and posture. Chedre seldom sees patients for more than fifteen sessions and has no trouble admitting failure, but he doesn't fail very often. In over 70 percent of the cases I have sent him, he has produced excellent results.

Profile of a Healer/Chiropractor. This chapter would not be complete if it did not describe a certain lovely type of chiropractor. Anyone who has met one of these will instantly recognize the type: the practitioner aged seventy or older who, through native gift and long practice, has reached beyond the technique of spinal manipulation to touch the essence of true healing craft. It was a chiropractor of this variety who inspired Dr. Chedre to choose his career. Many other superior D.C.s I have known were similarly kindled to excellence by such a role model.

When I knew Dr. Randall, he worked out of his home and charged only eight dollars per visit. He had cured a patient of mine named Gary, a young man whose football injury continued to give him terrible neck pain and headaches for more than five years. I wanted to know how he had done it, so I took Dr. Randall out to lunch. The chiropractor's explanation has much to teach about the higher forms of bodywork.

"When I put my hands on Gary's neck," he explained, "I could feel the injury all knotted up inside him, tied up as tight as five years of pain could make it. Underneath, I could sense the twist and turn that linebacker had given him. There were a lot of other injuries on top, but way inside, there it was, still trying to twist and turn. I don't mean that you could see it. You could just feel a kind of turn when you touched his neck.

"With all those years of pain, he'd tied knots in his knots. I'd have to untie them first, before I could get down to business. First three sessions I worked like the devil trying to peel away the layers. It made him hurt worse and he almost quit coming. But there wasn't any way around it. Finally, by the fourth visit, I was ready to work on the original injury.

"So I took this young man's head and gave it a gentle turn in the direction it was trying to go already. That's the way to let a body heal itself. You can't always fight a problem directly. Sometimes you have to kind of flow with it.

"I knew I was on the right track when I could feel that linebacker, with all his muscle and gristle, barreling right into that young man, and into me too. Not literally, you understand. I'm talking about something you feel when you listen hard enough with your fingers. Like a distant echo.

"The patient felt something too. All of a sudden he started sweating. He turned red, and moaned, and said it hurt all over. So I took the concussion of that linebacker and rolled with it just a hair, and held his neck in that position for about ten, fifteen minutes.

"To look at it from the outside, I hadn't done much to him. Just turned his head a little. But when that young man got up from the table, he looked real bad. I knew right then that I had either killed him or fixed him. He staggered out. The next day he called me. 'Dr. Randall,' he said, 'I'm sore all over, head to foot. I feel bruised. I haven't felt this bad for five years. What did you do to me?' I asked him to come right in.

"He *was* sore all over. Almost too sore to touch. I put my hands on him again that day, and what do you know? That turning and twisting was half gone, maybe three-quarters gone. His own body had done it. I held him there again, making a few slight movements—very gently, not fighting the injury, but going along with it. Two more sessions did it, and then it happened: that old phone call we all love to get. He said, 'Dr. Randall,' I don't hurt anymore. Five years of pain and this is the first time I don't hurt. I don't know what you did, but I'm glad.'

"That's the healing power of the body for you! It made him sore as heck on the way to curing him. Anyone who works with nature—feeling the life in people, not just tinkering with nuts and bolts—anyone who works like I do will tell you the same thing. The healing power of the body is fierce stuff."

A chiropractor doesn't have to be as intuitively gifted as Dr. Randall to make a difference. But when I make referrals for chiropractic, I always select professionals in whose heart lives the ideal of profound healing art, an ideal that only talent and long practice can bring to fruition.

MOVEMENT THERAPIES

All the bodywork arts discussed thus far involve the structure and function of the body as it lies, sits, or stands in place. But our bodies seldom remain still, even when we are sleeping. The movement therapies are methods of dealing with the body as it actually functions in motion. As a group, they can be quite helpful for chronic pain conditions that can be relieved briefly by other methods but quickly return.

The principal representatives of this category are Rolfing Movement Integration, Hellerwork, Pilates, Laban, Trager, the Alexander technique, and the Feldenkrais method. I shall focus most of my attention on Feldenkrais because it is by far the most widely available of these useful methods.

Rolfing Movement Integration and Hellerwork

Although the original system designed by Ida Rolfe was an essentially static modality, later practitioners realized the need to include movement retraining. Joseph Heller was a former Rolfer who designed the movement education program that bears his name. Subsequently, the Rolf Institute developed its own movement training program.

These methods have much the same uses as Feldenkrais, although they are somewhat less sophisticated. They teach proper movement through correction, observation, and conscious intention, whereas Feldenkrais accesses deeper levels of body awareness.

Pilates

Pilates is an increasingly popular system of exercise and movement retraining that dates back to early this century. Joseph Pilates was a teacher of Jack LaLanne and the developer of one of the first physical culture techniques. For many years his work was primarily used by dancers, but lately it has grown in popularity among the general public. The Pilates method involves special exercise equipment and techniques for improving the body's structure and function. It is more sophisticated than most physical therapy exercise systems and can be quite effective as a support to other forms of bodywork.

Laban

Rudolf Laban was a movement specialist who collaborated with Joseph Pilates. He spent many years studying healthy human movement and even developed a notational system for recording physical actions, used especially in dance. Laban had two profound insights about movement that have been influential in the subsequent development of all the important movement therapies. The first is that the human body tends to move in all three dimensions at once, making use of actions that seem superfluous but are actually essential for proper function. This subject is discussed further in the discussion of Feldenkrais.

Laban's other discovery began with the observation that infants go through a series of stages on their way to achieving an upright walk. He reasoned that when adults move incorrectly, they can rediscover healthy movement by retracing the infant's original steps.

When used as a therapy, Laban involves sequential activities based on normal childhood development. It is unfortunate that this important technique is not more widely available.

Trager

Milton Trager, M.D., invented a unique form of bodywork that uses gentle rhythmic rocking of the neck, trunk, and limbs. It produces a feeling of lightness and fluidity that can be remarkable. I personally find it more successfully relaxing than massage. However, I have seldom observed the Trager method treating any moderate to severe pain conditions.

The Alexander Technique

This is a highly aesthetic approach to movement work that is not for everyone. The Alexander teacher uses visualizations and gentle touch to help the student identify unconscious postural habits. As unhealthy habits are made conscious, they are deliberately altered to promote increased comfort, fluidity, and balance.

A certified Alexander teacher has completed sixteen hundred hours of training, and must be regarded as a sophisticated professional. However, the method is very subtle, and in my experience it produces good results only in those whose physical symptoms are relatively mild to begin with. Feldenkrais (as described below) seems to be effective in more advanced conditions.

Feldenkrais

The Feldenkrais method is another sophisticated bodywork form, a twin pinnacle alongside Rolfing. Moishe Feldenkrais, a physicist, was a contemporary of Ida Rolfe. It is said that of all the bodyworkers alive at the time, these great founders respected only each other. The techniques they developed are different but complementary.

Whereas Rolfe concentrated on the power of the fascia to influence the structure of the body, Feldenkrais devoted his attention to the systems that integrate and control body movement. In this dynamic mesh of nerves, muscles, and bone, he found another explanation to the puzzling question, "Why do I still hurt after all this time?"

This is a question I am asked frequently. Patients who have injured a shoulder, neck, or back want to know why they continue to hurt years later. Wounds in the skin heal within weeks. Fractures of the bone knit in months. It is reasonable, then, to wonder why injuries to the muscles and tendons persist for years. In the overwhelming majority of these cases, no cause can be seen on X ray, but the pain persists.

There is no easy answer to this question. Medical doctors generally believe that the tendons and ligaments of the neck and back simply do not heal well because their blood supply is poor. Another theory relates continued back pain to microscopic injuries of the intervertebral disks. Yet another assigns blame to scar tissue in the muscles. None of these theories has been demonstrated to be the major cause of prolonged pain, nor is any universally accepted as true.

An irritating school of thought among some medical doctors claims that chronic pain is just a disorder of brain chemistry, similar to depression. This is a rationalization for the famous line, "It's all in your head," and a justification for indiscriminate prescriptions of anti-depressants.

While there is no doubt that the brain plays a role in all illnesses, to claim that chronic pain is due only to low serotonin levels is to badly oversimplify the situation. There is obviously much more to chronic pain than mere altered mental perception. Doctors' instincts to the contrary, just because no damage shows up on X-ray, it doesn't mean that "everything is OK." The cause of pain's persistence has not yet been identified by present technology, but the pain is real.

Outside of the conventional realm, each branch of alternative medicine has its own explanation for prolonged pain. Chiropractors speak of spinal fixations; massage therapists of calcifications; and Rolfers of fascial disorganization. I am sure that all these conventional and alternative explanations capture part of the truth. Yet, the systems model promoted by practitioners of the Feldenkrais method is the one analysis that most impresses me for its insight.

According to Feldenkrais theory, the muscles, nerves, and bones of the body form an active and dynamic webwork of tissues. They function as an integrated system, somewhat like a computer network. Chronic pain is seen from this point of view as a system problem, a dysfunction in a network. This means that it is not so much individual bone spurs or muscle tears that are to blame for pain, although they might contribute to it, but a breakdown in the harmonious interwoven movements of linked muscle groups. This lack of harmony causes chronic discomfort and sudden spasms that seem to come out of nowhere.

Computer networks provide a convenient analogy. A large structure of interlinked computers can fail, not because of a fault in an individual computer, but because the whole system has fallen into a dysfunctional pattern. A computer network is supposed to function like a well-choreographed ballet. All the different parts are meant to mesh smoothly, forming a whole that is greater than the sum of the parts. But things can go haywire. Packets of information sent down the lines can get out of sync and begin to collide with one another. More and more work may go to certain parts of the system instead of being shared equally. A computer network can come to the brink of collapse without a single element of that network being damaged.

If there is enough reserve capacity available, an out-of-kilter computer network can continue to limp on for quite a while, manifesting only slower response time. But when there is a stressor, such as too many people signing on at the same time, the system can collapse. The computer network will then "lock-up" or "crash," sometimes with disastrous results.

The human body is similar to such a network, except that it consists of bone, muscle, and nerve instead of silicon and wires. To maintain the body upright or in motion, a complex pattern of opposing muscle groups pull against each other in

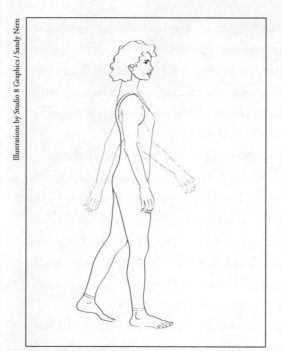

Figure 7.5 Walking in an upright position involves three-dimensional movements.

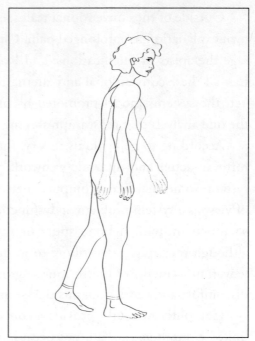

Figure 7.6 Injury can cause a person to walk leaning slightly forward with inhibited movement.

all three dimensions. Every movement involves a finely detailed sequencing of contraction and relaxation moving wavelike from muscle to muscle, and involves many muscles besides the ones seemingly at work.

For example, when people in good physical condition walk down the street, they invariably swing their arms. If you look closely you will notice that the arms don't swing stiffly forward and back. Rather, they move in three dimensions. They rotate, lift and drop, bend at the elbow and move toward and away from the side of the body.

It was Rudolf Laban's insight that these lively, three-dimensional movements are not performed just for show. Rather, they are necessary to ensure the continued health of the musculoskeletal system. Remember the old-fashioned barber sharpening his razor? He stropped it in an exuberant figure-eight motion. His was the right way to move; if instead he had scraped the razor back and forth like a robot, he would have developed a repetitive stress injury. The human musculoskeletal system needs to use complex movements to function properly. It is part of the normal functioning of the network.

But when people are injured, they develop inhibited patterns of movement. These begin as a natural impulse to minimize pain. People whose backs are injured may walk leaning forward; if their necks hurt, they may hold them rigidly to one side; if their shoulders are painful, they may raise them almost to the ears to reduce discomfort.

These are all natural and healthy responses to injury. Just as Rolfe noticed that distorted fascia can maintain improper posture, Feldenkrais realized that when an injury resolves, subtly altered patterns of motion may persist as new habits. For example, people may continue to move their arms stiffly back and forth even when their shoulder injuries are gone. They got used to moving that way while they hurt, and now that they are better they continue to walk like robots.

Emotional stress, work-related postures, and simple bad habits can do the same: create a situation where the web of movement pervading the body is inhibited and out of perfect sync. The body will try to compensate. As in the computer network that is out of sync, some muscles may perform extra work to make up for others that are doing nothing. But the body won't feel right. There may be chronic pain, a sense of fatigue, or simply a restricted ability to move. These symptoms are the physical equivalent of a slowing computer network approaching a crash.

Then, if a sudden wrong movement occurs, or a mildly incorrect position is retained for too long, a spasm may come on, seemingly out of nowhere. Many people complain about this, saying, "All I did was reach to the side and pick up a book," or "I just stepped off a curb." The reaction seems unfairly catastrophic for the apparent cause. But the cause had actually built up over a long time; the final spasm was only the culmination of a series of unnoticed changes.

According to Feldenkrais, systemwide movement problems are a major reason why pain persists and recurs long after an injury should have healed. The Feldenkrais method is a sophisticated system of movement reeducation that aims at restoring healthy movement patterns.

It was Feldenkrais's insight that mere exercise and postural retraining often fail to help. He observed that people unconsciously tend to use their strengths to cover up their weaknesses; in other words, they only exercise the muscles that are overactive already. Feldenkrais practitioners work subtly to overcome this obstacle. They increase their clients' awareness of movement, and focus their minds on the small nuances that make a big difference.

How Well Does Feldenkrais Work? While the above explanation of prolonged pain sounds wonderful and makes sense, what really matters is whether the treatment based on that explanation actually works. Here as in many areas of alternative medicine, there is nothing in the way of research information to serve as an objective guide. Clinical experience is the only available source of knowledge.

In my many years of working with Feldenkrais practitioners, I have seen the Feldenkrais method provide permanent relief in many cases of chronic or recurrent muscular pain. The success rate varies with the skill of the practitioner, the severity of the problem, and the patients' motivation to carry out the recommended exercises. Putting every case together, I would gauge Feldenkrais's effectiveness at roughly 50 percent, which is pretty good since most people turn to the slow process of Feldenkrais only when their problems are so severe that all other methods have failed.

In any case, Feldenkrais offers little in the way of instant gratification. This is a technique that takes a considerable investment of time to bear fruit. When Feldenkrais finally begins to succeed, however, the results are often long-lasting. Those who receive many sessions become so proficient at movement and so resilient that they are not hurt easily in the future.

How to Use Feldenkrais Therapy. I recommend that patients first try chiropractic and/or acupuncture as treatments for pain, because these methods produce quicker relief. However, if pain still persists after these methods have been given a full try, or if pain returns swiftly after treatment, then Feldenkrais may offer hope of a deeper cure.

Feldenkrais is available in two forms. The most inexpensive is the group lesson format known as Awareness Through Movement, or ATM. This educational process can be generally helpful, but it is not usually powerful enough to treat moderate to severe chronic pain. For such problems, the second form of Feldenkrais is most useful. This is the one-on-one therapeutic method known as

Functional Integration (in reference to its intention to work with function rather than structure).

It is difficult to describe what actually happens during a Feldenkrais Functional Integration session. The movement retraining is not so much oral as experiential, and it is not easily put into words. The Feldenkrais practitioner has learned to be highly sensitive to the unspoken language of the body, and can communicate in a way that bypasses the intellect, going straight to the unconscious levels where movement is organized. This is accomplished through directed passive movement, techniques that involve simple tools such as rollers under the feet, and focused awareness on movements that are already taking place unconsciously, among other methods.

Feldenkrais Functional Integration should be continued for at least twenty sessions before judging whether or not the treatment is going to be successful. This is a much longer waiting period than acupuncture or chiropractic requires. It takes quite a bit of money to discover whether or not Feldenkrais will help, which is why this treatment is best reserved for difficult cases.

After ten or more Feldenkrais Functional Integration sessions, it may be worthwhile to return for a few more acupuncture or chiropractic sessions, or to try Rolfing. The methods are all complementary, although Feldenkrais practitioners sometimes disapprove of chiropractic as being too rough.

However, it is difficult to combine standard physical therapy with Feldenkrais. Their recommendations tend to contradict one another. Feldenkrais practitioners take exception to many of the exercises conventional physical therapists recommend.

One interesting feature of Feldenkrais is that sessions can be tailored to fit the movement demands of real-life situations. I remember the amusing case of Martha, a professional bassoonist who came to see the Feldenkrais therapist with whom I shared an office. Martha suffered from neck pain during performances. Neither chiropractic nor acupuncture had helped her, so on my recommendation she tried Feldenkrais.

Barbara, the Feldenkrais practitioner, began by working with Martha's general movement skills. After about ten sessions, she decided it would be better if

Martha actually held the bassoon during the sessions. The two of them worked together in this way for several weeks. Still there was no improvement.

Success was not achieved until Martha actually *played* the bassoon while Barbara worked on her. It was only the stress of blowing into the mouthpiece and reading music that brought out the significant dysfunctional movement patterns.

After ten of these realistic sessions, Martha's problem disappeared. A side benefit was the bassoon concert to which my patients and I were treated every Thursday afternoon. (At first Barbara only asked her to play scales, but I found that dull. Nothing less than a full recital would stop me from complaining. It reproduced the real-life situation better, too.)

Will Insurance Pay for It? There is no specific license available for a Feldenkrais practitioner. In order to legally touch people for a fee, most obtain massage therapist licenses. Unfortunately, insurance companies therefore view treatments performed by Feldenkrais practitioners as high-priced massages.

A few Feldenkrais practitioners are physical or occupational therapists who grew frustrated with the limitations of their profession and felt a need to learn more. Insurance companies may be more willing to cover these practitioners.

Unfortunately, physical therapists who later become Feldenkrais practitioners are sometimes somewhat less skillful than those without previous conventional medical training. The modes of thought used in Feldenkrais are so different from the linear models taught in physical therapy school that some physical therapists are held back by their former habits.

How to Find Qualified Feldenkrais Practitioners. One virtue of this field is that most Feldenkrais practitioners are rather good at what they do. The Feldenkrais training program is rigorous, extensive, and brilliantly designed. However, it is not for everyone.

As a rule, successful Feldenkrais practitioners are not verbal, "left-brained" individuals. They enjoy focusing on details of movement to an extent that would bore most people to suicide. In the Feldenkrais training program of eight hundred or more hours, students participate in such fascinating processes as rotating their own left shoulders for sixty minutes at a stretch. The purpose of repetitive exercises like these is to develop intense experiential awareness of every nuance of movement. Most graduates of Feldenkrais training develop a sophisticated under-standing of human movement.

But, because they are so "right-brained," some of the best Feldenkrais practi-tioners seem a bit "spacey." They may also lack a mature business sense. These qualities do not speak against their skill in the practice of Feldenkrais; indeed, the reverse may be true. A person who is highly verbal and "left-brained" may not be able to slow down enough to practice the subtle arts of movement reeducation.

Finally, as is the case with other difficult crafts (such as playing the bassoon), Feldenkrais practitioners mature with time. A Feldenkrais therapist just out of training is not as good as one who has practiced for many years.

CRANIAL OSTEOPATHY

With the wide range of treatments covered by chiropractic, massage, and the movement therapies, it might be difficult to believe that another form of body-work substantially different from any of these could exist. Nonetheless, cranial osteopathy truly stands in a class all its own. This remarkable healing art is diffi-cult to practice effectively, but in the hands of a competent practitioner it is both useful and sublime. Amy Gilman's story illustrates its power.

It didn't require any great diagnostic genius on my part to guess Amy's com-plaint. When this twenty-eight-year-old mother of two took her seat before me, my own head ached just to look at her. Both of her eyes were partly closed, her neck was inclined forward and to the left, and her head rested on the fingers touching her left temple. She looked like someone had just struck her a blow to the skull.

In a slow, indistinct voice, Amy Gilman told me her story. Two years earlier she had been inventory supervisor at a large paper manufacturing plant. Her job entailed walking about various warehouses and checking stored materials. One day, while speaking to one of her subordinates, a piece of overloaded shelving col-lapsed, unleashing a cascade of steel drums. She jumped back, but not quickly enough. One of the drums struck her a glancing blow on the head.

Although she didn't lose consciousness, Amy saw a bright flash of light and fell to the ground. She tried to regain her feet in a moment, but her head throbbed so powerfully that she lay down again. An ambulance took her to the hospital for an emergency CT (computerized tomography) scan of the head.

The scan showed nothing, nor did a follow-up MRI a week later. Nonetheless, she could barely walk for the pain in her head. Amy's life came to a crashing halt. She couldn't work, take care of her children, or carry out basic household chores.

Because she had been injured at work, Amy's case fell under the auspices of worker's compensation. A claim was opened on her behalf, and she was granted temporary disability benefits.

Over the next two months Amy's head pain improved to the point that it was only disabling every other day; on the off days it subsided to a dull ache. Her doctors, encouraged by this progress, predicted that the headaches would soon go away altogether.

But they did not go away. At six months Amy still hurt too much to go back to work. Various follow-up tests came back uniformly negative. Her doctors tried every headache medication available, but nothing worked other than strong narcotics. These she avoided as a matter of principle. At one year postinjury, worker's compensation closed her claim. "You're well now," the case manager said.

Despite being officially well, Amy still hurt too badly to return to her job. Realizing that conventional medicine could not help her, she turned to alternative medicine. By the time she came to my office she had already tried chiropractic, acupuncture, herbs, food supplements, and massage. None of these had helped her. "Is there anything left to try?" she asked me, trying to smile.

Although I often find myself in the position of last resort, it is a responsibility I have never learned to carry easily. Too often I have nothing to offer. In this case, however, I knew what to recommend. Amy's injury and subsequent symptoms were a classic indication for cranial osteopathy, otherwise known as craniosacral therapy, or just "cranial" for short.

The nearest office of a competent practitioner of cranial was sixty miles away. It took some doing and help with logistical arrangements, but I managed to talk Amy into trying a series of sessions. After ten treatments she felt so much better she willingly signed on for another ten. At the end of the second series she was entirely cured.

What Is Cranial Osteopathy?

Cranial is a little-known but exquisitely refined form of bodywork. Properly performed, it is one of the most mature of the healing arts. It achieves a balance of subtlety and pragmatism that is rarely equaled in alternative medicine.

As the name implies, cranial osteopathy is an outgrowth of the larger field of osteopathic medicine. Founded by Dr. Andrew Still (1828–1917) in the late 1800s, osteopathy was a system of medicine that grew to be a strong influence on all subsequent alternative medical practice in the United States.

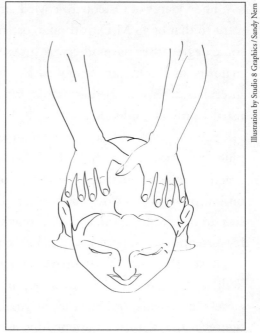

Illustration by Studio 8 Graphics / Sandy Nern

Figure 7.7 Cranial osteopathy uses subtle movements.

Dr. Still believed that health was sustained by the free flow of fluids and nerve impulses through the body. He regarded disease as the result of obstructions to that flow. To restore health, it was necessary to remove such obstructions. Dr. Still invented various forms of manipulation to accomplish that goal.

The fundamental osteopathic methods are called articulatory techniques. These are similar to chiropractic manipulation but applied to all joints of the body. Indeed, chiropractic itself is essentially an offshoot of Still's work, but osteopathic medicine does not make the spine so central an issue. Other common osteopathic methods include myofascial release and muscle energy manipulation, as discussed earlier in this chapter under the heading of massage.

Unlike the founders of chiropractic, the leaders of osteopathic medicine formed a strategic alliance with medical doctors at the beginning of the twentieth century. This led at first to a flourishing of osteopathic colleges and practitioners, but, ultimately, to a partial loss of identity. By now, osteopathic medicine has virtually been assimilated into the larger stream of conventional medicine.

The Doctor of Osteopathic Medicine degree (D.O.) is presently legally equivalent to that of an M.D. Although osteopathic colleges still teach manipulation to some degree, they have otherwise grown quite similar to medical schools. The vast majority of D.O.s are simply M.D.s by another name. They may be surgeons, internists, allergists, or dermatologists. If they still perform manipulation, it is usually only as a sideline.

Some doctors of osteopathy retain a primary allegiance to the original philosophies espoused by Dr. Still. They perform manipulation as a large part of their practice, sometimes at high levels of competence. Many individuals aware of the option prefer to visit osteopaths over chiropractors, because osteopathy has never succumbed to the commercialism that so plagues chiropractic. However, relatively few osteopaths can perform spinal manipulation as well as excellent chiropractors.

A small group of osteopaths practice cranial osteopathy, the invention of William Sutherland, D.O. In my opinion, these dedicated practitioners come the closest to actualizing Dr. Still's original vision. Dr. Sutherland was an important figure in the history of osteopathy, as well as in American alternative medicine generally. By all accounts, he was remarkable for his ethics, his authenticity, and his steady, patient work. Entirely lacking flash, sparkle, or untoward charisma, he attained little fame but left a deep mark on those who knew him.

It was while attending osteopathic school in Missouri that Sutherland made his celebrated conceptual leap. He had been studying a human skull "disarticulated" into its several bones. The edges of the bones where they connected to one another caught his attention. These "sutures" are strangely beveled in such a way as if to permit a bit of movement. Yet, according to the conventional wisdom of medicine, the bones of the skull should be fixed and immobile. Could it be that they did move?

Sutherland speculated that perhaps the skull expands and contracts, like the lungs. This rhythmic motion might pump, not air, but the clear cerebrospinal fluid that surrounds the brain and spinal cord. Fired by his idea, Sutherland embarked on a systematic study of the skull. He found that the bones of the cranium do undergo a definite rhythmic rocking; a swivel and rotation too slight to be seen but detectable by careful palpation. He named this rhythmic movement the cranial rhythm. Sutherland believed that this movement extended the full length of the spine, producing a related pumping movement in the sacrum—hence the longer name, "craniosacral."

Sutherland theorized that the force behind this pulsation originated in the tissue containing the cerebrospinal fluid—the dural sac. To the whole complex of moving bones, sac, and fluid he gave the title "the primary respiratory mechanism" (or "the mechanism" for short).

After perfecting his ability to detect this cadenced pumping action, Sutherland examined patients suffering from various diseases. He observed that in many of them the normal pattern of movement seemed blocked or irregular. Following the general principles of osteopathy, he theorized that blockages to the cranial rhythm could be an important cause of illnesses.

Next, Dr. Sutherland developed techniques for restoring normal movement of the mechanism. He found that by gently manipulating the bones of the head and sacrum he could produce relief from many symptoms. Sutherland called his method "osteopathy in the cranial field" to acknowledge his debt to classical osteopathy.

Is the Cranial Rhythm Real?

The cranial rhythm Sutherland described is very slight. Only with practice and great concentration can it be perceived at all. A cranial practitioner observes it by placing his hands on the skull and feeling for a subtle rise and fall occurring at intervals somewhat further spaced than the breath. An untrained observer cannot sense it.

The natural question arises: If only cranial practitioners can feel it, how can we be sure that the cranial pulsation exists? Perhaps Sutherland, for all his integrity, simply suffered from delusions. Indeed, until recently, the only evidence for the rhythm's existence was the word of cranial osteopaths. Numerous attempts to scientifically verify the existence of this rhythm through objective means failed to produce concrete results. This should not be surprising, for it was cranial practitioners who performed those experiments. Technology was simply not the natural bent of these healing artists.

In the world of conventional medicine, however, this lack of objective research meant that Sutherland's conclusions were entirely disregarded. Most medical doctors still believe that the bones of the skull do not move. As for the grandly titled primary respiratory mechanism, virtually no scientist outside of osteopathic medicine has even heard of it.

Part of this situation is beginning to change. Definitive evidence establishing the existence of the cranial rhythm has been produced at last and published in prestigious journals. Numerous medical doctors throughout the world have performed corroborating experiments showing that Sutherland was right: the bones of the skull do move in a slight but definitive regular undulation. Whether this rhythmic pulsation is as fundamental to health as Sutherland believed, however, remains unclear.

A Glimpse into Cranial Osteopathy

I was introduced to the cranial technique by a fellow holistic physician. Intrigued by her description, I enrolled in a forty-hour workshop sponsored by the Cranial Academy of Indianapolis.

The Cranial Academy is the most serious of all organizations dedicated to the teaching of cranial osteopathy. Its active members are almost like priests of William Sutherland, so devoted are they to a man whom they regard as a historic figure. Greatly concerned to maintain a high standard of excellence, and fearing that if the art is disseminated to nonphysicians it will degenerate, the academy allows only D.O.s and M.D.s to attend its retreats.

Most of the teachers at the seminar I attended wore bow ties and black suits. They behaved formally, although not stiffly, and carried in their persons a whiff of the graciousness of another era. When they spoke, it was nineteenth-century medicine come back to life. Compared to modern medical doctors, these osteopaths appeared quaint, colorful, dreamy, and reverent—distinctly premodern in their manner and thinking.

They spoke of William Sutherland and Andrew Still with warm reverence. At each session they recited the principles of osteopathic medicine almost as a catechism, and the students were requested to join in. The lecturers told stories with fervor and a sense of the miraculous, qualities absent from conventional medical gatherings.

The Cranial Academy puts great stress on precise anatomical details. This emphasis is important, I believe, because it gives solidity to what is otherwise a very subtle treatment method. Cranial practitioners who know little of the anatomy involved tend to regard what they do as a form of "New Age energy work." Not so with members of the Cranial Academy. They insist absolutely that they are working with a concrete physical process, not an airy-fairy concept.

Much of the workshop was occupied with studying the movements of the bones of the skull. The cranial bones are complexly three-dimensional and their spatial relationships hard to visualize. To understand the movements of the cranial mechanism, it is essential to grasp precisely how each bone rotates, swivels, and slides against the others.

To assist in the learning process, every table was supplied with two skulls: one intact, the other disarticulated (separated at the sutures). With furrowed foreheads and overloaded fingers, we students propped the tiny pieces together and attempted to re-create each movement. We spent at least twelve hours racking our brains to understand the precise movements of the mechanism.

Finally, most of us mastered the rudiments of the essential anatomy. The speakers then advanced to the art of palpation. Placing our hands gently on the heads of fellow students, we closed our eyes and concentrated intensely on the in-and-out rhythm we had just studied. Some students felt it immediately; others could not perceive any movement for hours. And then, suddenly, aha! I believe I learned to feel it too, although I cannot tell for certain whether it was just my imagination.

The Signature of a Healing Art

I came away impressed by the sense that cranial treatment is a mature healing art. Through my experiences with many forms of alternative medicine, I have come to consider certain characteristics as the universal signature of healing in depth. Cranial bears this stamp.

All those who work closely with the liveliness of living things seem to share a common language. Psychotherapists, gifted bodyworkers, dancers, athletic coaches, bonsai gardeners, organizers, old-fashioned chiropractors like Dr. Randall, portrayed earlier in this chapter—all these seem to me to converge toward a certain essential understanding of the nature of healing. Cranial puts this orientation into the most physical of terms.

For example, cranial practitioners stress that simply "following the rhythm," or allowing the hands to feel the ebb and flow, is therapeutic in itself. This is strikingly reminiscent of a view held by Rogerian psychotherapy (named for Carl Rogers): that concentrated attention heals.

In a further similarity to the techniques of psychotherapists, cranial osteopaths seldom apply force to directly correct an abnormality. Their theory states that direct action is relatively ineffective. The body will tend to resist a head-on confrontation with its patterns, and try to reinstate a pathology that has become the norm. Rather than engage in a hopeless struggle, the cranial osteopath encourages the body to move still further in the pathological direction toward which it is already moving. The practitioner holds the body in a position of exaggerated imbalance for several minutes. Finally, when the body itself tires of maintaining so extreme a posture, it voluntarily initiates a recoil toward normalcy. (Dr. Randall used the same method.)

This process echoes closely the amplification techniques used in many schools of psychotherapy. In these methods, the therapist deliberately intensifies the client's psychological patterns. The client is held at a point of maximum experience, until the pattern releases spontaneously. For example, a man who is angry at his father may be encouraged to shout "I hate you, Dad" for an entire therapeutic hour, until at last he falls down, exhausted, ready to make peace.

At heart, the same process is used when a community organizer decides to treat gang leaders with respect, realizing that it is not direct opposition, but affirmation and sensitivity, that will produce successful results.

Cranial therapy also bears a distinct similarity to creative arts such as dance. Both use nonliteral metaphors to describe what they are doing. For example, osteopaths speak of "feeling two inches past the fingers." This is not a reference to magical or psychic gifts. Rather, it is a metaphorical use of language necessitated by the subtlety of the processes involved. The movements of cranial manipulation are so small, and the adjustments so delicate that concrete terminology is inadequate. "Feeling past the fingertips" means contacting tissues that cannot be touched directly, using the subtle clues communicated through intermediary tissues.

A dancer once used similar words when describing to me the method she used to keep in rhythm during a complex line dance. "I feel the movements of the leader, pulsating through the hand of my partner," she said, even though she stood four bodies distant in the human chain. This is a form of useful poetry, not a statement of literal fact.

Thus, while cranial osteopathy is not "energy work," its methods are so refined they cross over from mere mechanics into realms of profound art. Only a few branches of alternative medicine equal its subtlety.

Portrait of a Cranial Osteopath

After attending the cranial seminar, I gave some thought to incorporating cranial therapy into my practice. To this end, I obtained permission to observe and assist in the office of Dr. Ralph Houston. He was (and is) a classic osteopathic physician of the old school. Among all the cures I have seen produced by practitioners of alternative medicine, his have most impressed me for their depth and apparent ease.

Dr. Houston's appearance was unimpressive. He wore an old tweed coat, and his shoes were of an outdated style. His hands, however, stood out like tended roses in an alley—slender, sensitive, and strong. Dr. Houston carried his hands as if they were crown jewels.

Unlike conventional medicine, where younger doctors are often more proficient than are older ones, long experience counts most in cranial osteopathy. Dr. Houston had practiced nothing but cranial osteopathy five or six days a week for forty years. He was regarded as a master by others in the profession.

Dr. Houston treated two patients each hour. Punctually, at five minutes before the hour and half-hour, he would walk upstairs to record his chart notes. In session, he talked constantly while his fingers worked. His surprising stories drew his patients' minds into reveries conducive to healing.

My favorite story was the one he told about a young woman injured in a fall from a ladder. The force had driven her left leg into her pelvis and twisted her neck backward and to the right. After a little traction, her skeleton looked normal again, but she suffered from terrible back pain. When Dr. Houston put his hands on her, he could feel the force of her injury throbbing and pulsating beneath his fingers. His best efforts, however, could not bring about a release. Twenty treatments had produced no results. He was near the point of giving up.

Then, on the way to her twenty-first visit, the woman's compact car was totaled by a full-sized pickup. Feeling that she now needed him more than ever, she managed to reach Dr. Houston's office at the appointed time. He put his hands on her and, to his surprise, discovered that the original injury had vanished. He asked her how she felt. "Why, come to think of it," she replied, "I feel better than I have in years." The force of the impact had served as a perfect correction to her original problem!

According to the old osteopath, this proved that "God is the real healer, not us humans." Whatever they may have believed themselves, the effect of this story, like so many others he told, was to draw Dr. Houston's patients into a state of mind where "the world is known to be filled with healing power."

Meanwhile, Dr. Houston's hands sought their work. His fingers moved about their business with a refinement and sensitivity contrasting sharply with the appearance of the man to whom they belonged. Although Houston did not appear to concentrate on the bodywork, his interventions proceeded with great skill. His experiential knowledge of the interconnections of the human body had grown so deep as to become instinctive.

When Dr. Houston cradled the skull, patients would report sensations in the back, feet, pelvis, and abdomen. He would hold his hands still for a minute, then gradually release contact, removing his hands far apart in a graceful gesture. At times he would work on the sacrum, the chest, or the feet, initiating movements too slight to see, but productive of far-flung results. A pain might appear, grow to excruciating levels, then subside; a memory of past injury might arise; an emotion, a cramp, a twitch could develop in an instant and just as instantly dissolve.

He credited the power of his minuscule interventions to the cranial rhythm.

"Because it drives the whole body, when I synchronize with it my fingers carry a force that is not my own. I could literally lift a patient off the table with my fingertips, if I did it right, but it wouldn't really be me doing it. The rhythm provides the power and the timing. I ride along the wave of the mechanism, pushing just a little. You can tear apart a bridge if you find its resonant frequency. This is the same idea."

The most dramatic immediate effect of his work was the process known as unwinding. (A similar process is seen in other forms of bodywork.) As Dr. Houston exaggerated the imbalances he felt beneath his fingertips, patients would often undergo bizarre spontaneous movements. These might involve serpentine motions of the trunk, or rapid, rough jerks shaking a limb or the whole body. Over the course of several sessions these spontaneous postures would first increase, then level off, and finally fade away entirely. When the unwinding was complete, the patient often reported dramatic reduction of symptoms.

In Dr. Houstons's office I saw many cures of disabling, intractable headaches, tailbone pain, backaches, and neckaches. Because I shared several patients with the osteopath, I was able to verify that these cures were real and long-lasting.

I have never been so impressed by the relative frequency of a healer's successes as I was with Dr. Houston. Furthermore, the healing seemed to occur at a deep level. Once cured, patients were not dependent on further treatments. Symptom relief was profound and stable.

Other Cranial Practitioners

After observing Dr. Houston, I gave up on the notion of providing cranial therapy myself. I lack the ability to focus for long hours on body sensations. Unfortunately, I have often found it difficult to find qualified cranial practitioners for my patients.

Dr. Houston himself maintains a fourteen-month waiting list. Only about one thousand osteopaths are listed by the Cranial Academy as qualified practitioners of cranial osteopathy. To discover these names, contact the Cranial Academy at the address listed in the Resources section at the end of this book.

An osteopathic physician named John Upledger gives seminars to the general public on his variation of cranial therapy. Unfortunately, I have been relatively unimpressed by the skills of many who have taken his training.

There is also a chiropractic version of craniosacral called S.O.T. (sacral-occipital technique), but it lacks entirely the subtlety of true cranial work. Some acupuncturists have studied cranial therapy, following the example of the brilliant acupuncturist/osteopath Dan Bensky, but few practice it regularly enough to develop real competence.

If I can find no cranial practitioner near enough to treat a patient, I may recommend Feldenkrais instead. Of all bodyworkers, Feldenkrais practitioners alone seem to possess equivalent depth and sensitivity.

Sensitive bodywork is a rare skill, especially in America. A technique that requires an ability to concentrate on delicate tactile sensations runs counter to Western cultural trends. Americans are, generally, left-brained, active, interventive, and intellectual. Yet cranial is a homegrown art. By rights, it ought to be an Eastern healing form, like the art of Shiatsu practiced by Japanese blind people. It amazes me that the same level of skill lives here in the West, among old-fashioned osteopaths, bow ties and all.

What Is Cranial Osteopathy Good For?

The major usefulness of cranial osteopathy lies in the condition known as post-traumatic headache. This is the severe, intransigent head pain that sometimes follows concussions and other severe blows to the head. Responding poorly to medication, this type of headache may continue for many years, as it did for Amy Gilman. In my experience, cranial osteopathy offers the greatest likelihood of cure. Twenty or more sessions may be necessary for full treatment.

Cranial is also useful for problems caused by blows to the tailbone. According to theory, the tailbone is the bottom pole of "the mechanism." It too is supposed to move rhythmically with the pulsations of the cerebrospinal fluid. Experientially, many people who fall on their tailbones develop severe headaches. The cranial technique can be useful for this problem as well as for pain in the tailbone and sacrum itself. I have also found cranial osteopathy to be useful for neck pain, back pain, and temporomandibular joint pain.

Practitioners of cranial osteopathy go much further in their expectations than the few conditions I have just described. They believe that they can cure a wide variety of other health problems, including frequent sinus infections, misaligned teeth, scoliosis, mental illness, and others. However, it has not been my experience that cranial actually works very well for any of these ailments.

Dangers of Cranial Osteopathy

Occasionally a very sensitive individual will develop headaches or some other adverse reaction in response to cranial osteopathy, but such events are rare and nearly always short-lived. Cranial osteopathy is simply too delicate a technique to cause direct physical harm. When performed incorrectly it simply does not work.

But, like all other forms of alternative medicine, cranial presents a risk to the pocketbook. Treatment can go on forever without success. I recommend stopping treatment after about ten to twenty sessions if there is no result.

In case of treatment failure, I suggest trying one of the other bodywork arts. This category of treatment is so broad and diverse that among its many methods a patient is likely to find a modality that can succeed.

CHAPTER 8

Body / Mind Medicine

There is no longer any question that the mind influences the body. Study after study has shown the power of stress to worsen virtually every illness, and "stress-related illness" has become a term in common use. But conventional medicine instinctively shies away from dealing with mental and emotional influences on health for the usual reason: these factors are too fuzzy and subjective for medical doctors' comfort. Therefore, the subject has largely fallen into the alternative camp.

Most every alternative practitioner gives some attention to the meeting of body and mind. Some advocate methods of reducing stress such as meditation, yoga, or guided visualizations. Others focus on positive mental attitude and its power to improve well-being, or teach the use of visualizations to combat cancer and other diseases. Methods such as these can complement other conventional and alternative techniques.

This subject is taken one step deeper by practitioners of the "body-oriented" schools of psychotherapy, such as Hakomi and Process Work. According to these schools, hidden or blocked aspects of the total self are fundamental to illness.

Another influential approach to the subject comes from the world of spiritual seekers, whether Christian, Buddhist, or New Age.

One important characteristic of body/mind approaches is that they are valuable in their own right regardless of their effects on a particular illness. They are capable of promoting an increased sense of overall well-being and an enhanced experience of life.

A full treatment of body/mind interaction is beyond the scope of this book. However, I briefly introduce the subject here because it is such a ubiquitous part of the alternative medicine landscape.

STRESS REDUCTION

Randy Thompson is perhaps the most dramatic case of healing through reducing stress that I have ever encountered. While his story is exceptional, it illustrates beyond any doubt the power of the mind to influence health.

In the late 1970s Randy had been a successful restaurateur, owning six restaurants in a major market. His workload had soared along with his fortunes. By 1982 he was earning a million dollars profit a year, but his duties kept him busy more than ninety hours a week. He enjoyed the challenges of business and, if asked, he would have said that he thrived on the stress.

Then he fell ill with multiple sclerosis (MS). Unlike the typical slow progression of this disease, in Randy's case the symptoms came on rapidly and inexorably, leaving him wheelchair-bound within six months. He rapidly lost the ability to manage his work and was forced to sell his restaurants.

At this point, Randy took an unusual step: he became a hippie. Actually, it had been his secret dream for some time. He had often toyed with the idea of taking up the freewheeling life of a social dropout. But this was the early 1980s, and Randy had to reinvent hippiedom practically from scratch. He searched long and hard to find living examples on which to model himself. Considering it an appropriate first step, he bought a used Volkswagen van and fixed it up with a wheelchair lift and other accommodations to his illness. Then he drove around the country, staying in campgrounds, listening to street musicians, and generally avoiding all deadlines, pressures, and responsibilities.

Not only did he enjoy himself tremendously, Randy's MS symptoms began to subside. Within a year he could walk again; within two, he was in better physical shape than ever before. He climbed mountains, played the guitar, camped by the ocean, and attended Rainbow-People gatherings, always making sure to stay relaxed.

After five years of this happy life, an inner voice began to nudge him toward working hard again. "You have no excuse," it said. "You're not sick anymore. Don't you think you should be making money?" Obeying this prompting, Randy bought a restaurant.

He found the return to productivity enjoyable, and he was still good at his work. Within a year his restaurant was a thriving establishment. He was about to open another when his MS started to come back.

Randy had no trouble getting the message, but it took him time to get out from his new responsibilities. By the time he had completely disentangled himself, he was back in a wheelchair. Fortunately, after only a year of hippie life again, he completely recovered.

Not everyone has the means to so thoroughly escape from stress, nor would becoming a hippie help every MS sufferer. I tell the story not as a specific recommendation but to illustrate that stress reduction can be a powerful influence toward improved health. Time pressures and constant crises produce a continual fight-or-flight response that exhausts the system. Many illnesses improve when stress levels are reduced. Everyone agrees on this, but the question is what to do about it.

Numerous methods can be useful for diminishing the harmful effects of stress. Besides retreating from modern life, some of the most famous techniques to cope with its tensions are meditation, yoga, guided visualizations, biofeedback, and regular aerobic exercise.

Of course, stress reduction methods must be actually practiced to produce good results, and practiced diligently. Some of the most stressed-out people I have ever met teach stress reduction courses.

MEDITATION

Meditation has many forms, from the primarily spiritual approach of Zen Buddhism to completely secular techniques such as autogenic training. Most employ some form of concentration on the breath and methods to teach "letting go" of anxieties and extraneous concerns.

Meditation instruction is often available at local community centers. As always, some instructors are much better than others. The TM (transcendental meditation) program offers a systematic approach to meditation, but its methods are not particularly better than others, and they may be more expensive. Numerous books are available on the subject, each of which will appeal to different individuals.

YOGA

Hatha yoga is a traditional exercise form from India, used to promote meditational states of awareness through the disciplined use of the body. It is also traditionally believed to produce a variety of health benefits directly. Anyone who has tried it knows that the regular practice of yoga can create a relaxed body and mind.

Many types of yoga are taught in this country. The best focus considerable emphasis on the breath. Some forms of yoga are excessively athletic and should probably be avoided except for the purpose of developing unusual physical skills. Kundalini and other "energy raising" forms of yoga are only for those who wish to pursue yoga as a spiritual approach to life. Yoga for the purpose of relaxation is only generically spiritual; its concentration is on peacefulness rather than specific beliefs.

Yoga should never be learned from a book or a videotape. A person who is habitually tense will tend to perform stretching exercises tensely unless a teacher is present to provide correction. I have treated many people who were harmed by self-taught yoga.

Yoga courses are widely available in most communities. As always, the level of proficiency of the instructors varies widely.

GUIDED VISUALIZATION

This is a form of meditation that makes use of visual imagery led by a therapist. Typically, the therapist begins by making simple suggestions that promote relaxation, such as advising the client to deliberately relax each major muscle group. Next, the therapist tells a simple story and invites the client to imaginatively enter into it. A typical story describes a walk that leads out of a stressful city environment and ends up in a secluded natural scene.

Those who are visually oriented may find this form of meditation easier than traditional methods. Guided visualizations can also be used in a more active form; in that case they are sometimes called positive visualizations, described later.

BIOFEEDBACK

Biofeedback is the most scientifically respectable method of promoting relaxation. The technique is based on the discovery that human beings have the capacity to learn to influence elements of their bodies that previously were under automatic control.

For example, few untrained individuals can deliberately affect their heart rate at will, but almost everyone can learn to do so. All that is necessary is a mechanism that gives direct information about the speed of the heart: in other words, a source of feedback about a biological state, or biofeedback for short. A simple meter that displays heart rate is sufficient. Through looking at the display and wishing the heart rate to raise or lower, most people can with practice become able to control the speed of their heart. Thus, a previously automatic bodily function can be brought under conscious control.

This method can be extended to allow deliberate control of practically any body function. The practical use of biofeedback is to keep the body in a state of relaxation even when it is under stress. Biofeedback training is widely available, often under the auspices of a psychologist.

POSITIVE THINKING

The concept of positive thinking was popularized early this century by the New Thought movements. From the Church of Religious Science and the Unity Church to Emmet Fox and Norman Vincent Peale, all proposed some variation of a singular notion: the cause of illness is negative thinking. Recent proponents of the same idea have included such notables as O. Carl Simonton, Deepak Chopra, Werner Erhardt, and Jane Roberts's channeled entity "Seth."

According to one version of this philosophy, the proper method to deal with illness is to deny that it exists. Proponents of this approach recommend affirmations such as, "I am perfect as my Father made me perfect, whole within and without." Another variation permits a sense of improvement, such as the famous mantra, "Every day, in every way, I am getting better and better."

The method of positive visualization is similar. Popularized by O. Carl Simonton as a treatment for cancer, this technique involves conjuring up images of friendly soldiers shooting at cancer cells, and so on. There is some evidence that such methods can improve survival if performed vigorously.

The growing science of psychoneuroimmunology has begun to elucidate the actual biochemical means by which mental processes can influence virtually every event that goes on inside the body, although much more remains to be discovered.

Again, there are innumerable books on the subject, and a number of practitioners who teach methods from this repertoire. What are required for success are self-discipline and a natural ability to harness the mind. Stories abound of incredible cures through mental concentration, and I am sure that many of them are real.

Some individuals find these methods easy to use. But others find themselves absolutely unable to think positive thoughts no matter how hard they try. For them, the doctrine of positive thinking can become a trap. I have known many sick people who have made themselves sicker this way. The first step in the downward spiral is the thought, "I must have created my illness by thinking negative thoughts." Then comes the realization: "But I think negatively all the time. Therefore I must be constantly creating new illnesses for myself. I wonder what terrible disease will strike me next?" Next, the Catch-22: "But look what I'm doing right now! I'm predicting that I will get sick. That's more negative think-

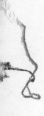

ing." It circles around again: "I'm sure to get sick if I keep worrying about it. Oh no! That's a negative thought. I'm doing it again!"

This trap is surprisingly common, and those who promote positive attitudes seldom warn against it. Some people simply cannot help looking at the dark side. By leading them to believe that this habit will in itself make them sick, the doctrine of positive thinking becomes a source of despair rather than of healing. I counsel such people to adopt an altogether different philosophy, such as the classic "Learn to feel what you are actually feeling" of psychotherapy, or the "Turn it over to your Higher Power" of Alcoholics Anonymous.

BODY-ORIENTED PSYCHOTHERAPY

Stress reduction and positive thinking are fairly simplistic approaches to the body/mind interaction. Out of the immense complexity of human emotional reality, they focus on only a few fixed concepts. The schools of depth psychotherapy that study physical symptoms examine the subject more profoundly.

The belief that physical illnesses may be connected to deep inner processes is an ancient one. In religious circles, it has always been believed that unforgiveness or other unconfessed sin may eat at a person from within. Sigmund Freud expressed the same belief using the new language of psychology when he attributed physical illness to repressed emotion. Carl Jung felt that symptoms could represent lost parts of the inner self asking to be incorporated into the whole.

All these views and more are used by the body-oriented psychotherapies in their search for psychological healings of physical illnesses. Approaches influenced by Wilhelm Reich use stressful body postures to induce "releases" of frozen emotion. Author Louise Hay interprets illnesses as messages from the body, often couched in the form of puns. For example, if a person has neck pain it might indicate he is too "stiff-necked" in the psychological sense.

Arnold Mindell's process-oriented psychotherapy takes the subject a step further. Like Jung, Mindell regards physical symptoms as parts of the true self wanting expression. In his words, "A terrifying symptom is usually your greatest dream trying to come true." From a process-oriented point of view, Randy Thompson recovered from MS not so much because he reduced stress but because becoming a hippie actualized a deep desire of his heart.

Mindell views illnesses as "dreams in the body." He explains that just as hidden parts of the self express themselves in dreams, they may also manifest as body symptoms. Mindell believes that by discovering and welcoming these pieces of potential personality, the need for a physical symptom may diminish, and the patient may get better. His approach to facilitating this integration is called process work.

One patient of mine provides a great example of process work in action. Katy came to me complaining of interstitial cystitis. Medical treatment had failed her and she wanted an alternative approach. Interstitial cystitis is a chronic illness of unknown cause. Among other symptoms, it involves a continual sensation of the need to urinate in the absence of a bladder infection. Conventional medical treatment can be painful and expensive, and unfortunately only temporarily successful.

Katy had already endured three invasive procedures. During the initial interview, I began to suspect that her circumstances were ideal for an application of Mindell's techniques. This proved to be a fortuitous guess. Katy's story proceeded exactly "by the book." I do not want to leave the impression that deep healing usually occurs as easily as it did for her. Most real-life situations are complex and intertwined, and the outcome far more murky. However, simple cases make the point most clearly, and that is why I often retell Katy's story.

To begin the work, I asked Katy to describe her symptoms subjectively. She hesitated a moment, then explained, "Well, it feels like a pressure demanding to be let out!"

"Does it have a color?" I continued. It did not. "How about a motion?" Katy replied that it did, and spontaneously demonstrated the motion by moving her arms repeatedly away from her body, palms forward, fingers spread out, as if she were pushing against a resistant barrier.

"Could you amplify the movement you are making?" I asked, following Mindell's method. "Be this pressure. Be the symptom, as if you were a symptom having a body, rather than a body having the symptom." This embodying of a distressing symptom allows more information to express itself.

Katy understood. She stood up and pressed vigorously against the invisible obstacle. I became a cheerleader. "Really be the symptom, Katy," I said. "Move as much as you like. Make noise. Let yourself into it."

She began to utter irritable noises and grunts that soon turned into words. "Let me out of here, let me get out of here right now!"

"Yes, what you are saying is just right," I encouraged. "You want to be let out. Go on!" It is an important part of the technique that the therapist does not introduce interpretations, but merely reflects what is emerging on its own.

Suddenly Katy stopped, with an amazed look on her face. "I know what it's about!"

If I had been looking for intellectual meaning, I would have asked to hear her insight. But Mindell's method does not primarily seek an analysis of a problem. It seeks the inner self hidden in the problem. Mindell emphasizes that purely cognitive understandings seldom produce as much actual change as an experience realized in bodily feeling.

"Don't think about it yet, if you can avoid it," I cautioned. "Perform it. Express it. Act it out."

She pondered the best way to express her realization. Not wanting to give her an opportunity to think too much, I kept pushing. "Just go for it. Don't make plans. Let your realization speak in actions. Let the process express itself."

Katy paused for a moment, then broke through. "Let me out of here! I'm tired of being in here. I'm tired of waiting, of being so civilized, of acting like a proper lady." As she spoke, Katy hooked her thumbs in her belt loops and swaggered, doing a fair imitation of a female gunslinger.

I encouraged her to amplify the role further. She walked up to me and pushed me on the shoulder. "Listen when I talk to you, Bub. I'm not in the habit of letting men like you tell me what to do. I'll do what I want, when I damn want it."

Although I knew we were only play-acting, I actually felt personally intimidated by her fierce face and confident manner. I stammered out a submissive "Yes, ma'm," which was more sincere than therapeutic.

Katy looked radiant. Recovering my role, I suggested that she drink in the sense of confidence she felt. "Allow it to penetrate your body. Allow it to permeate your life." Only after she had fully absorbed the feelings the role-playing had created did I ask to hear her insight.

"I am absolutely sick and tired of being the nice little girl I was raised to be," she explained. "I always act like that—at work and at home. It's the real me that wants to get out!"

When she returned the following week, Katy had many stories to tell. At work, she had started to speak up for her own ideas. Surprisingly, her supervisors had responded well to the new assertiveness. Katy had been taken aside twice, not to receive a rebuke, but to be praised for her intelligence and forcefulness. At home it was a different story. "But, if my husband doesn't get with the program, he can be replaced!" she laughed.

Over the next month, Katy's urinary urgency decreased and finally disappeared. One session of process work was sufficient. Her medical condition has never returned to its original strength, although it flares up from time to time when she turns aside from her new path.

This story is a classic and almost too-perfect example of psychological issues manifesting as physical symptoms. Katy had spent thousands of dollars on crude and painful medical procedures that entirely missed the point. Rather than surgical interventions, what she needed was to express in real life the part of her inner self that the symptoms represented; a part symbolized by a tough, low-life female gunslinger.

It was not so much Katy's intellectual realization that helped her as it was the emotional force behind it. After all, the personality development she was prompted to undergo is a very familiar one. Many women are working on some variation of the "discovering one's power" motif. Anyone could have told Katy from the outset what she needed to do; in fact, she had often given herself the same advice. What is different about the methodology of process work is that through amplification the actual force behind the symptom is harnessed to produce personal growth. The interstitial cystitis was not a mere message. It *was* her personal power striving to emerge.

As one of Mindell's students put it to me, "Behind every symptom is a powerful natural force. If that force can be accepted and put to use, it will change the topography of a person's life."

Those who study with Arnold Mindell sometimes seem to think that nearly all diseases are metaphorical. This is a natural exaggeration. In my experience, while I would agree that useful and growth-promoting metaphors may be derived from most diseases, only occasionally will that effort relieve the original symptoms. Katy was lucky.

SPIRITUAL APPROACHES

Many spiritual approaches to healing touch on the body/mind connection. Examples include Christian faith healing, the Buddhist-inspired approach of Stephen Levine, Christian Science, New Age spirituality, Native American spirituality, and Scientology. Depth Jungian psychology can probably be regarded as a spiritual approach as well. I mention the subject here only for completeness, for it is outside the scope of this book. Any large bookstore stocks numerous volumes on the subject.

HOW WELL DO BODY/MIND APPROACHES WORK?

In my experience these forms of healing require considerable commitment to succeed. A dab of stress reduction combined with a positive visualization or two will avail nothing. Those I have known who really benefited from body/mind methods first chose a method and then fully immersed themselves in it.

Unlike most other approaches to healing, however, this method is useful in itself. While taking dietary supplements or receiving chiropractic treatment may relieve a particular problem, doing so is not particularly ennobling or broadening. But body/mind methods have the capacity to enrich the whole life of the one who undertakes to try them.

SECTION IV

HOW TO USE
ALTERNATIVE MEDICINE

Conventional medicine has spoiled us by providing standardized protocols and statistical information on which to make choices. As the preceding pages have shown, little of the kind is available in alternative medicine. Successful use of alternative methods requires persistent effort, the patience for extended trial and error, and the ability to make decisions based more on "gut sense" than on hard facts.

In these requirements alternative medicine resembles nothing so much as life in general. Most day-to-day decisions require similar skills. There are no established protocols for choosing a mate, a job, or a place to live. Individuals can identify useful alternative therapies and competent practitioners with no more or less difficulty than they can navigate other arenas of life.

This section provides practical hints with the aim of making these admittedly complex choices a bit easier.

CHAPTER 9

General Principles

When I first became interested in alternative medicine, I made numerous errors of judgment. Everyone must make their own mistakes, but this chapter attempts to communicate a few principles I discovered over those years of trial and error.

GUIDING PRINCIPLES

Persist Through Trial and Error

Above all, alternative medicine is a learn-by-doing affair. No one makes it through the jungle of alternative treatments without taking many wrong turns and wasting a fair amount of money. With experience comes the ability to make more informed decisions.

Don't be afraid to switch practitioners and methods. Often, the worst practitioners and the shallowest methods possess the most persuasive advertising. While it is easy to be taken in by a salesperson, it takes time to learn to recognize true quality.

Avoid New Methods

Alternative medicine is bedeviled by faddism. I make it a rule to ignore all newly minted methods for at least five, preferably ten years. Science has made us fans of new discoveries, but alternative medicine doesn't work the same way. Would you expect to find new discoveries in cabinetmaking or pottery? Because alternative medicine consists primarily of crafts whose efficacy depends more on skill than on brilliant new insights, "new" is not necessarily the same as "better."

New discoveries *can* be significant in the more scientific aspects of alternative medicine. For example, the uses of food supplements and herbal extracts are constantly evolving. However, practitioners of alternative medicine seldom take a cautious wait-and-see attitude toward early research results. They tend to base treatments on results that can barely be described as preliminary.

Most supposed breakthroughs in alternative medicine are just new pyramid marketing schemes. Since one year's magic cure-all is usually pushed out by the next one, I suggest waiting a while. Time tends to scathe away nonsense. If a product or methodology stays around for a decade, it is more likely to have something to offer.

Avoid Overly Simple Solutions

While we would all like to find an easy answer to our health problems, life is seldom so simple. Every year one or two books come out proposing a delightfully easy answer to a great variety of health problems. Whether it's juicing, eliminating yeast, or chasing away parasites, simplistic solutions like these seldom work, except to line the pockets of their originators.

Look for maturity and humility in alternative medical advice. Sophisticated practitioners understand that health and illness are complex subjects, and that every method has its limitations.

Learn to Recognize Integrity and Ability

Some alternative practitioners are better than others. The same may be said of entire alternative methods. Excellence can be identified by research, recommendation, and referral, but most important is your own ability to discriminate. Use the same skills you would use to evaluate a potential employee, roommate, or carpenter.

Don't Be Too Impressed by Testimonials

Every method, healing philosophy, and product has its glowing testimonials. Some of these are even true. I have met people apparently cured of asthma by vitamin B6; of cancer by the Gerson diet; and of emphysema by a Mexican arsenic product. But because a method works stunningly for one person does not prove that it is a powerful cure for the masses.

Emotionally, it seems that if a method produces dramatic results even once, it should be a marvelous breakthrough that will cure nearly everyone of the same condition. But strangely enough, it isn't so. It is a fact of life in alternative medicine that many methods work wonderfully once or twice, provide mediocre results occasionally, and fail most of the time. I could recite hundreds of examples. The overwhelming majority of miracle cures work for only a small minority of the people who try them.

It is more cost-effective to use methods that stand a fair chance of succeeding at the outset. These are rarely marketed by testimonial, but rather by long tradition or solid science. In Section V, I try to indicate the most useful approaches for a variety of common conditions. In my experience, however, even the best of alternative methods seldom succeed more than half the time. Conventional medicine has spoiled us again in this regard, by providing many methods that work 70 percent of the time or more. Nonetheless, even a 40 or 50 percent chance of success is far better than nothing.

Trust Your Own Experience

Most often, the only laboratory in which to test alternative medicine is your own body. Pay attention to results. Often, a few treatments will give an indication whether a method is going to work. Don't be afraid to follow "gut-feelings" and intuition. They are often your best guide.

Just Because It Makes Sense
Doesn't Mean It's True

Many alternative theories sound nice on paper but don't really work. I have learned this the hard way by falling in love with innumerable health beliefs and preaching them to friends and relatives before fully trying them out. Each one seemed to make sense at the time.

For example, early in my involvement with alternative medicine I became enamored of the idea of fasting. A little booklet I picked up at a natural food store promised that fasting would "cause the body to eliminate all the toxins of disease." I liked the sound of it, and intuitively felt it was true. Enthusiastically, I embarked on a campaign of progressively more intensive fasts. Unfortunately, while this was a good experience in the development of willpower, it didn't make me any better—just very thin.

Next, I encountered the principles of homeopathy. Once more I was fascinated by the elegance and clarity of the theory. But this method too failed to help me.

I was not a quick learner. At least twenty times I was seduced by elegant health theories before I at last discovered what I should have known all along: Theories are just theories. What works in real life is another story.

In my experience, the more perfect-sounding the theory, the worse the practical results. Pragmatic approaches to healing are like clothes that have been mended a hundred times: they are full of patches to cover holes in theory, and patches to cover the holes in the patches to the theory. Real healing is an intensely practical affair.

Don't Rule Out a Practitioner
Just Because He or She Has a Few Faults

This concept too has been hard for me to grasp. It used to be that if I caught a healer smoking in the back room, or sneaking ice cream at the Häagen-Dazs store, I would disown him as a hypocrite. If he showed a commercial streak, I would write him off as a charlatan. If he said many things I knew to be untrue, I would consider him a fool.

Only with time did I discover that such strict requirements would eliminate practically every practitioner of alternative medicine. The field must be approached more forgivingly. Nonsense and value are closely intermingled in all the branches of alternative medicine. Even the best alternative approaches are partly baloney!

The best practitioners of healing arts are often badly flawed in one way or another. I used to refer patients to a chiropractor who spent every session spouting a continual stream of half-baked theories and praising himself to the sky. Despite all the nonsense, he was one of the most skilled spinal manipulators I have ever met. I simply told patients I sent to him to stop their ears with plugs before opening his door.

Don't Fall in Love with a Healer

There is an apparently universal human inclination for hero worship. On the slightest shreds of evidence, we will lionize someone as a step above ordinary mortals.

I have done this myself when I was a patient, and have had it done to me many times since I became a doctor. Louise comes to mind, a patient who believed that I was an all-powerful alternative healer. By sheerest luck, and after several false starts, I had managed to cure her of terrible migraine headaches. But to this day I don't know why the method I finally used helped her. Acupuncture had failed, Chinese herbs had done nothing, and my referral to an excellent chiropractor had made her worse. Then I recommended feverfew, a famous herbal treatment for migraines. I had little confidence in this recommendation because Louise's headaches seemed too serious. But when I ran out of other options I finally mentioned it.

To my astonishment, the feverfew provoked an extraordinary series of symptoms racing through her body in quick succession. Louise sweated, vomited, suffered partial paralysis, fainted, dreamt horrid dreams, and developed the worst headache of her life. Then, most extraordinary of all, her headaches disappeared and never returned.

Feverfew is not supposed to behave this way. Its usual effect is to alleviate a given migraine, and possibly to prevent future ones if taken consistently. But Louise took it four times and never needed it again. I have never seen feverfew work this way, and it probably never will again.

This lucky happenstance made Louise my fervent admirer. She told all her friends how marvelous I was, thereby setting me up to disappoint most of them.

Excessive faith like this is a common occurrence. When alternative practitioners succeed once or twice they are then imagined to be miraculous healers. Some may regard this as a fortunate opportunity to make use of the placebo effect, but I personally don't like to participate in wishful fantasies.

In truth, no one really knows much about healing. All healers are groping in the dark; able to help at times, often failing, sometimes making people worse. This is true of every branch of medicine, from brain surgery to shamanism.

CHAPTER 10

Common Questions about Alternative Medicine

The patient who seeks alternative medical care immediately faces several difficult practical questions: What kind of problems is alternative medicine good for? How should I pick a particular practitioner? Do I put myself in any danger by making this choice? Can I get insurance coverage? How can I get my M.D. to make a referral to an alternative medicine practitioner? This chapter attempts to provide answers, insofar as it is possible to do so.

WHAT KIND OF PROBLEMS IS ALTERNATIVE MEDICINE BEST FOR?

Chronic pain is the most obvious indication for alternative medicine. Beyond providing the valuable service of ruling out potentially dangerous causes, conventional medicine typically has little to offer for pain. Fortunately, many branches of alternative medicine are rich in offerings for various pain conditions—most notably acupuncture and all forms of bodywork.

Alternative medicine may also be quite helpful in the treatment of general symptoms such as malaise, fatigue, and inability to concentrate. Again, it can be very important to have a conventional doctor rule out serious problems. But if all the tests come out negative, it is time to try alternative medicine.

Another good indication for alternative medicine is the problem I call "metadiseases." By this term I refer to a high frequency of recurrence of an otherwise treatable or self-limited disease: in other words, too many sinus infections, frequent sprained ankles, recurrent yeast infections, and the like. While conventional medicine may be able to treat each individual occurrence of these problems, it can seldom lower the frequency of recurrences. Alternative medicine may be able to come to the rescue.

Actually, most mild to moderate problems will respond to some form of alternative treatment. Where there is a high risk of death or permanent injury, however, alternative medicine is probably not appropriate. An old story goes: If the electrical insulation in a house becomes frayed, it should be fixed expeditiously. If it is not repaired in time, a fire may result. Once a fire starts, however, it is too late to work on the insulation. It is time to call the fire department.

Alternative medicine tends to be far better at replacing insulation than at putting out fires. The time for alternative treatment is early, before the situation gets out of hand. Once there have been several heart attacks, multiple hospitalizations, or repeat surgeries, the value of alternative medicine is considerably diminished.

See section V for recommendations on alternative treatments for specific conditions.

HOW SHOULD I CHOOSE
AN ALTERNATIVE MEDICINE PRACTITIONER?

This can be a difficult problem, but no more so than finding a good auto mechanic or a carpenter. What is necessary is an informed referral.

One of the best referral sources is a professional in a related field. Just as an auto body repairman can usually recommend a good mechanic, and vice versa, one kind of alternative practitioner can often recommend a good one of another type. Chiropractors often know the best acupuncturists in town, and vice versa. Health food stores are also good sources of referrals.

Friends will often recommend their favorite practitioners, but before taking such advice it is essential to make sure that the friend has seen more than one practitioner. Someone who has visited many different acupuncturists may be able to give informed advice as to which one is most skillful; but a person who has been to only one or two will not have developed any comparative standards.

Although there are no precise indications that can demonstrate the relative competence of an alternative practitioner, common sense can provide some general tips. For example, it is better when practitioners are fully trained in their skills and show an ongoing interest in continuing education. Therefore an acupuncturist with two thousand hours of training and a long list of postgraduate seminars should be preferred over a medical doctor who has taken only a weekend course in acupuncture.

Another useful guideline is years in practice. Alternative practitioners of all varieties tend to improve with time and experience. Those just out of training tend to be naively optimistic.

I personally prefer practitioners who are humble and ready to admit the possibility of failure. These qualities show maturity of character. I have to admit, however, that many highly skilled practitioners are remarkably arrogant. There are no hard-and-fast rules here, and no substitute for a well-developed sense of discrimination.

Shop around and experiment. The skills required to evaluate an alternative medicine practitioner develop with practice. It takes experience to distinguish true confidence from hype, skill from bluster, depth from fantasy, and genuine talent from good marketing skills.

IS ALTERNATIVE MEDICINE DANGEROUS?

Those who are opposed to unconventional treatment often warn of the serious dangers facing those who seek it. They make two major charges: that alternative medicine practitioners keep people away from receiving the medical care they need; and that alternative therapies can directly cause harm. This attitude, however, is based more on prejudice than on fact. In reality, little evidence exists of any grave danger to the public health posed by alternative medicine practitioners. Of course, one can always find individual horror stories, but the same can be said for conventional medicine also.

Probably the worst danger anyone faces when visiting an unconventional practitioner is financial. In other words, you may waste your money. An unscrupulous healer may sign you up for hundreds of visits that do not help you. Even a very scrupulous one may treat you with the best of intentions, but fail to improve your health.

Few studies have been performed to evaluate the success rates of alternative techniques. Therefore, practitioners may at times provide treatments that do not work. This does not necessarily involve fraud. Alternative providers may think they are doing something helpful, when it is only wishful thinking.

Common sense, however, suggests that a treatment that keeps attracting new customers for many years must have some value. Thus, chiropractic, with its hundred-year history, and acupuncture, which goes back thousands of years, very likely work at least sometimes. Otherwise, people would have stopped going to these practitioners long ago.

Medical doctors often fear that alternative health care providers keep patients away from legitimate medical treatment when they really need it. This can occur, but it is relatively infrequent. Alternative medicine practitioners are ordinarily afraid to talk their patients out of conventional medical treatment (or to tell them to stop their medications), for three reasons. One, they are afraid of lawsuits and bad publicity. Two, their license does not allow it. Three, most cases of genuine medical urgency are dramatic and frightening, under which circumstance most patients go to a regular doctor on their own.

A good rule of thumb might be as follows: If you are worried that you may have a serious health problem, do not allow an alternative medicine practitioner to lull you into complacency. Visit a medical doctor. Medical doctors are vastly better at diagnosing serious illnesses than anyone else; the skills of alternative practitioners are more properly utilized for treating chronic problems of a mild to moderate nature.

Of course, medical doctors may insist on treatments just out of habit, even when they really make no sense. It is generally advisable to be assertive with M.D.s and to demand clear explanations. Ask, "Why do I need this drug [test, surgery]?" Consider the doctor's explanation, and make your best decision.

The instances where the treatment provided by an alternative medical provider can actually harm a patient directly are relatively few. A chiropractor, through overly vigorous manipulation, can occasionally cause injury. An acupuncturist who is not careful may inadvertently puncture the lungs or a large blood vessel. A naturopath might prescribe dangerously high doses of vitamins.

In all these cases, the professional involved would have been trained in school to avoid these mistakes. Of course, he or she might still make an error.

It is quite common that an acupuncture, chiropractic, or massage treatment can temporarily worsen pain, but these problems are usually short-lived.

CAN I OBTAIN HEALTH INSURANCE COVERAGE FOR ALTERNATIVE MEDICINE?

Patients often ask me how they can obtain health insurance to cover alternative therapies. They have heard that alternative medicine is cost-effective, preventive, and far safer and more effective than conventional medicine. Therefore, insurance companies should flock to write policies to cover it.

While the insurance coverage for alternative medicine is gradually increasing, the process is much slower than advocates would prefer. This is not only because of stodginess on the part of insurers, but also because of more fundamental obstacles in the way of alternative health care insurance.

To understand these obstacles, it is first necessary to consider the nature of insurance. Insurance is meant to protect against unexpected catastrophes that the insured does everything in his or her power to prevent. For example, few people wish to be involved in automobile accidents, to have their houses burn down, or to die. Auto insurance, fire insurance, and life insurance are available to protect against these disasters, and policyholders hope they won't have to collect on their policies. When disaster does strike, money is made available to the victims from the pool of money provided by nonvictims.

However, standard health insurance fails to follow the insurance model fully. Only a hospitalization policy (the original form of health coverage) is truly a form of insurance. To be hospitalized is a relatively rare event that most people earnestly prefer to avoid. It is also most often out of the patient's control. Therefore, hospitalization can be insured against in much the same fashion as the types of insurance mentioned above.

Office medical practice is another story. Colds are neither rare nor catastrophic, but they do lead to office visits. Furthermore, patients and doctors have it in their power to determine how often office visits occur.

While hospitalization insurance parallels automobile accident insurance, general medical benefits are more like automobile repair insurance. Such insurance does not exist.

Consider the consequences of such hypothetical coverage: Car owners and mechanics would between them determine the need to put a car in the shop. Yet because they would not be paying repair costs themselves, car owners would care little about the expense. No doubt, certain car owners would bring their vehicles into the shop weekly to maintain the highest possible performance level. Mechanics would similarly recommend ever more frequent checkups to avoid being sued for unexpected automotive failures. Frequency of repair and costs per repair would spiral out of control.

Contrary to all the rules of insurance, consumers who purchased auto repair policies would plan to collect on their policies. They would purchase auto repair insurance with the express intention of saving money, hoping to pay less in premiums than they save in mechanics' bills.

But that is impossible. Insurers cannot pay out more in claims than they take in as premiums. They are not charities. To prevent unlimited cost escalation, third-party payers would have to develop strict rules for coverage. For example, they might restrict coverage for tuneups to every 20,000 miles or more. Repainting might be classified as cosmetic work and therefore excluded from coverage. The replacement of timing belts would only be covered for those owners who could document a taxilike driving pattern involving frequent stopping.

Automobile owners would find a thousand reasons to argue against these restrictions. Some might claim that their particular cars don't hold their tune-ups and need more frequent adjustments. Others would say that their cars need preventive repainting to avoid costly corrosion problems in the future. There would be no end to the arguments and special cases.

A bureaucracy of rules, inspectors, and rulemakers would spring into existence to control costs and validate legitimate exceptions. Mechanics and car owners would invent clever ways to get around the rules. Car maintenance organizations (CMOs) might spring into being, made up of mechanics who agreed to serve a certain pool of customers for a fixed total fee. (In HMO jargon, this is called "capitation.") This would lead to car repair rationing, as mechanics tried to do as little as possible for the money they were paid.

This fantasy, of course, exactly parallels the health care system as it exists today. Because medical care fails to follow a true insurance model, health insurance is necessarily byzantine.

But if conventional health care is problematic, the situation of insurance coverage for alternative care would be even worse. Even though it is not a catastrophe like a house fire or a hospitalization, it is generally at least a little unpleasant to visit a medical doctor's office. In contrast, many people truly enjoy alternative treatments. Just as car owners might want to take their cars in for weekly detailing and regular tune-ups, some individuals might want to get acupuncture, chiropractic, or massage every week, or even twice a week, just to feel good.

It is impossible to insure against events that people enjoy! A Blue Cross branch discovered this when it offered a pilot program in alternative medicine: Nearly everyone who signed up used their coverage to the limit. The experiment cost the company millions of dollars.

To cover alternative medicine, insurers would have to introduce numerous arbitrary limits. This is what has been done for chiropractic and psychotherapy: restrict coverage to, say, ten sessions a year. Unfortunately, it is difficult to imagine on what rational basis underwriters could design their rules. Nobody knows what works and what does not, nor how many treatments are necessary. Whatever rules could be designed would tend to be capricious, arbitrary, and insensitive to individual needs.

Some people claim that covering alternative care will save money for insurers in the long run, because it is so wonderfully cost-effective and preventive. Unfortunately, this is a romantic dream. Therapies such as chiropractic, massage, and acupuncture are labor-intensive and anything but cheap. Supplements aren't free either. Furthermore, it is often necessary to try many different types of alternative treatments before hitting on one that works, thereby multiplying the costs.

As far as prevention goes, the only truly cost-effective forms of prevention are those for which a patient does not need a doctor at all: namely, regular aerobic exercise and a semivegetarian diet. Few forms of alternative medicine prevent problems in themselves. Chiropractic, for example, treats neck and back pain well, but unless it is continued on a maintenance basis, the patient's back or neck will always "go out" again. And maintenance chiropractic is expensive.

What has been discussed so far does not exhaust the problems of alternative medicine health insurance. Consider the further question: What alternative care should be covered? Chiropractic, acupuncture, Rolfing, and nutritional counseling only? What about iridology? Chelation therapy? Laetrile? Shamanism? Macrobiotic education? Raw foods counseling? Who would set the standards and who would draw the lines?

For all these reasons, if blanket insurance coverage ever comes to include alternative medicine, it will not be the simple, happy event proponents envision. Currently, individual insurance companies are offering coverage for specific alternative therapies on a case-by-case basis, always making sure to charge more for the coverage than the average costs that will be incurred. No doubt the availability of such coverage will grow in response to consumer demand.

Whether such developments will actually be good for alternative medicine remains to be seen. I fear that some of the best qualities of the healing crafts may be injured by too close association with large insurance bureaucracies. Despite the problems, the medical model and the insurance model possess strong similarities. Both are based as much as possible on hard facts and objective data. It would be a loss if all healing arts were forced into the same rigid mode.

HOW CAN I OBTAIN REFERRALS TO ALTERNATIVE MEDICINE PRACTITIONERS?

Insurance companies will sometimes cover alternative treatment only if a medical doctor makes the referral. Obtaining such referrals can be quite difficult. For best results, a different strategy must be used for each type of alternative practitioner.

Conventional doctors have more experience with chiropractors than with any other form of alternative provider. Unfortunately, there is a long history of animosity between these professions. Another obstacle to referrals is the unfortunate reputation for commercialism that chiropractic has earned. Even doctors sympathetic to chiropractic feel uneasy about turning their patients over to practitioners for whom money may be a primary consideration.

Nonetheless, many physicians have developed good relationships with select chiropractors. A bit of time spent on the phone can often identify these doctors. Just ask the receptionist, "Does Dr._____ever make referrals to chiropractic?"

Physicians are usually much less prejudiced against massage therapists than against chiropractors. It is usually not hard to obtain a referral for therapeutic massage, although the medical doctor is not likely to successfully distinguish between the various branches of massage therapy. Generally, it is not a good idea to try to enlighten a physician on the nature of Rolfing or Hellerwork. Simply make sure the physician doesn't write the name of a specific massage therapist on the prescription. Just say you have your own.

Acupuncture as a treatment for pain also enjoys a fairly good reputation among physicians. Most doctors already recognize that conventional medicine has little to offer for pain treatment. Therefore, many do not object to authorizing a trial of acupuncture treatment, especially if the acupuncturist is another physician. (Unfortunately, physician-acupuncturists are seldom fully trained in the art as non-physician licensed acupuncturists.)

I suggest never discussing acupuncture treatment for conditions other than pain. Most doctors find the concept difficult to accept. Bringing up the subject will only tend to damage the patient's relationship with the physician.

Practically no physician has heard of Feldenkrais or any other movement therapies. In any case, even if a medical doctor did make such a referral, insurance would almost certainly not pay for it. The only exception is if the Feldenkrais practitioner is also a physical therapist, in which case treatment can be authorized as physical therapy. Simply ask the doctor to authorize physical therapy generically. The physician need not know that the physical therapist is actually practicing the Feldenkrais method.

Naturopathic practitioners present a special problem. Because naturopathy is the most nearly scientific of all forms of alternative medicine, it might seem that doctors would feel favorably disposed toward it. However, this is not the case in real life. Most doctors find naturopathy extremely offensive. It comes too close to home.

Acupuncture is so completely nonscientific that it doesn't "push any buttons." But because naturopathy frequently invokes science, its many flagrantly unscientific aspects irritate medical doctors. For this reason, in the few states in which naturopaths are licensed, it is usually difficult to find a physician who will make referrals to them. The most likely candidates are recent graduates of family practitioner residencies. These physicians are often surprisingly open-minded. Of course, naturopaths may already know a physician willing to make referrals to them.

Many other good questions can be asked regarding alternative medicine, and I encourage asking them. The field will only benefit from intelligent evaluations and thoughtful analysis.

CHAPTER 11

Integrating Conventional and Alternative Treatment

Ideally, conventional and alternative medicine should supplement one another. No approach to healing is so universally competent that it can address all health problems successfully. Patients need all the help that is available.

Unfortunately, the attitude of medical doctors toward alternative medicine is typically somewhat less enthusiastic than a warm embrace. Numerous patients have told me the same story: "I asked my doctor whether there wasn't something natural I could take, and what did he do? He slammed the chart down and walked out. Why don't doctors have open minds?"

The explanation is simple: Alternative medicine is not a neutral option; it passionately criticizes many aspects of conventional medicine. Like all human beings, medical doctors are attached to their own beliefs. They frequently respond to criticism with criticism of their own, usually in the form of blanket statements disparaging every aspect of alternative therapy.

Because of this intrinsic opposition, as well as for other reasons, conventional medicine has long used its prestige and authority to suppress alternative options. In recent years, however, the power and popularity of alternative medicine have increased. Some alternative proponents have begun to dream of a day when their work will be the dominant health care form. In my opinion, that day is still far off, if it is even in the cards at all. Alternative medicine remains far too immature and divided to replace the prevailing paradigm. Yet, a readjustment in relative positions is already in the works.

Other authors imagine that conventional and alternative medicine will eventually meld into one greatly expanded form of healing that combines the best of everything. Again I disagree. I believe there is a place for diversity in life. The world needs both civil engineers and ballet dancers; I wouldn't want to drive on a bridge designed by a ballet troupe, nor watch a crew of civil engineers dance to *The Nutcracker Suite*.

Similarly, the gifts of conventional and alternative medicine are equally significant but quite distinct. Rather than dissolving their boundaries and melting into oneness, it would be more useful for each to continue to develop in its own direction. The problem is not that the fields are different. What causes patients trouble is the lack of mutual respect.

Instead of learning to embrace fuzzy concepts, conventional practitioners should strengthen their devotion to precision and reproducibility. Accurate biomechanical medicine has made a tremendous contribution to health care and will continue to do so in the future. But scientific healers should acknowledge that the subjective healing arts have a contribution to make too. On the other side of the divide, practitioners of the healing arts should work to deepen their own healing gifts, while at the same time honoring the reliability of scientific knowledge.

Unfortunately, this day of mutual respect has not yet arrived, except in isolated pockets of harmony. As a general rule, conventional and alternative practitioners do not presently get along well. Therefore, it falls to patients to create their own integrated approach to health care. The information presented in this chapter is intended to assist in that creative and ongoing process.

DIAGNOSIS

One of conventional medicine's greatest strengths is diagnosis. Techniques such as the Pap smear, the MRI scan, and various blood tests can discover the presence of diseases long before their symptoms become evident. Of course, medical diagnosis isn't perfect. Every medical test results in a certain percentage of false calls. But there is simply nothing in alternative medicine that can compare.

Perhaps the most important use of diagnostic tests is in ruling out serious diseases such as cancer. In fact, medical doctors expect most of the tests they perform to come out negative. They perform them only for prudence' sake. It is often very useful to utilize conventional medicine's powers in this regard while at the same time turning to alternative medicine for treatment.

TREATMENT

For many conditions, alternative medicine is much better at treatment than conventional approaches. Chronic pain is the classic example. Even when there is an effective conventional option, it is generally appropriate to try alternative methods before resorting to drugs or surgery in all mild to moderate conditions. Every drug has its risks and all surgeries their dangers. In the overwhelming majority of cases, alternative options are far safer.

Conventional medicine is ordinarily preferable to alternative treatment in cases of illnesses that threaten death or serious injury. Nonetheless, alternative medicine can still sometimes play an auxiliary role in these conditions. For example, herbal treatment can often diminish a diabetic's need for insulin.

HARD FACTS

Conventional medicine is far more trustworthy on the level of hard facts than any branch of alternative medicine. If a medical doctor says that a patient has liver damage or that a given treatment holds out a 27 percent chance of success, it is likely that these statements are factually correct.

The speech of alternative providers, however, can seldom be trusted at a concrete level. Most are "right-brained" intuitive individuals, not "left-brained" precisionists. When a naturopath says, "Your adrenals are weak," these words may have no meaning in terms of literal fact. There may be nothing physically wrong with the adrenal glands. The expression "weak adrenals" is more a useful conceptual framework than a tangible reality.

Failing to realize this relative vagueness, patients often falsely suppose the naturopath's statement to be as concretely true as a medical doctor's. The concept of weak adrenals is a far vaguer one than the medical notion of "partial kidney failure," or "25 percent aortic regurgitation." Nonetheless, the naturopathic treatment for "weak adrenals" may be quite helpful.

Similarly, when acupuncturists say, "This herbal combination will help your rheumatoid arthritis," they mean they believe it will help, based on the tradition they have learned and what their clinical experience has taught them. They do not mean the herbs have been proved to work, nor that they have been tested in even a single study, nor that any objective data exist. Their sources of knowledge are "soft."

HEALING

Conventional medicine's pursuit of hard facts has given it a reliability that alternative medicine cannot match. At the same time this quest has made medicine ponderous, hidebound, slow to move, insensible of most finer feelings, and unaware of delicate touches. Scientific medicine is relatively soulless and mechanical.

Alternative practitioners, on the other hand, often develop deeply perceptive personalities. Their hands-on skills may be akin to those of a master carpenter or a world-renowned musician. Alternative medicine provides scope for the true spirit of healing to embody itself.

Some techniques are more congenial, more transparent to the outflow of healing intention than others. For example, few medical doctors are healers, some acupuncturists are healers, many bodyworkers are healers, and those who perform laying on of hands are healers or nothing, for their work has no technique to shroud or guide the inner goal.

NATURAL LEANINGS

All professionals have tendencies that, if understood, make it possible to evaluate the advice they give. If a surgeon recommends against surgery, that advice can probably be trusted. Conversely, if a chiropractor advises you to consider back surgery, I recommend taking that recommendation seriously. But when a surgeon advises surgery, or a chiropractor a long course of chiropractic, both may be reasonably suspected of self-serving behavior.

I recommend taking note of a practitioner's inclinations. When a medical suggestion goes against that grain, it is probably impartial and highly reliable. In other cases, a second or third opinion is advisable.

PARANOIA VERSUS TRUST

Conventional medicine is a profession of dread. Medical doctors are trained to look for any possibility, no matter how remote, that could pose a danger to a patient. Few alternative practitioners take on that responsibility. Instead, most adopt a positive, life-affirming, and faith-filled stance. They generously extend their trust to ancient healing traditions, the teachings of famous healers, their own intuitions, and the presumed power of the body to heal itself.

By contrast, conventional medical doctors are skeptical to the point of paranoia. Physicians expect to find the worst and constantly fear disaster. They practice maintaining "a high index of suspicion."

In modern times, few alternative practitioners have treated enough cases of serious illnesses to take illness seriously. But almost every medical doctor has stood through many disasters in a position of responsibility. Extremely respectful of the power of disease, they dread to miss a sign or ignore a symptom that, if noted, could stave off disaster. This constant state of alert is central to the practice of medicine, and is not just a result of malpractice suits. Scarcely one in a hundred alternative practitioners has the sense of mortality, the sense of responsibility, or the raw determination to save patients from disaster as do the least responsible of medical doctors.

Most patients understand this distinction. For this reason, alternative medicine practitioners are seldom sued. When they are used, expectations are seldom high to begin with. In contrast, medical doctors are supposed to be a perfect safety net, catching all those at risk of falling seriously ill. They are held accountable for every disease that slips through undiagnosed.

Both trust and anxiety are valuable. In reality, it is just as unreasonable to expect a medical doctor to provide constant positivity as it is to look for careful prudence among alternative practitioners. The two attitudes are almost mutually exclusive. This issue is so primary but so little understood, I believe it is worth devoting two long anecdotes to explaining it.

These stories come from my own practice. Because I attempt to offer both alternative and conventional medical services, I am forced into managing these two opposing roles at once. As a medical doctor I am expected to catch rare and dangerous diseases; as an alternative practitioner I am supposed to trust the healing powers of nature. It is seldom possible to do both well.

Andrea was a woman in her forties who came to see me for a feeling of chronic fatigue and a constant cough. She strongly disliked orthodox medicine, but she felt it was prudent to inquire whether she might have a serious condition. She had chosen me because I was an alternative doctor.

I hesitated before replying, because this is a tricky question, especially with patients who distrust conventional medicine. "What would be your preferred basis for a sense of safety?" I asked. "For example, I could tell you what my intuition says: Intuitively, I feel that you don't have anything serious."

Andrea smiled broadly. "Well, that's good to hear!"

"Don't get too excited," I cautioned. "That is only my intuition. I'm not always right." She frowned. "I could perform an examination according to the principles of Chinese medicine," I told her. We could investigate whether or not your energy seems dangerously out of balance."

She nodded enthusiastically.

"But I must tell you that I have no idea how often Chinese medicine is right. No one has ever done any studies on it. Honestly, I don't know if Chinese medicine is right 25 percent of the time, 50 percent of the time, or 90 percent of the time."

Andrea relapsed into a state of anxiety.

"We could do medical tests," I continued. "Medical tests are not 100 percent accurate, but the accuracy is at least known. Is this the route you want to go?"

Andrea replied slowly. "Well, I think if we do some tests, and they come back negative, I'll feel safer than before. What would you want to look for?"

I proceeded to list some of the diseases that could be causing her symptoms. Among other possibilities I mentioned anemia, low thyroid, asthma, hepatitis, Lyme disease, fibromyalgia, and rheumatoid arthritis. Then as an afterthought I asked whether she was a smoker.

To my surprise, Andrea said she was. This unexpected piece of information forced me to add the possibility of lung cancer, as well as emphysema. Noticing that my patient was no longer smiling, I quickly emphasized that she probably didn't have a single one of those conditions.

This provoked her. If she didn't have those problems, why was I wasting time talking about them?

I reminded Andrea that she had requested me to make sure she had nothing serious. In conventional medicine, that is done by ruling out all the relevant possibilities. Andrea finally agreed to take several tests.

I expected to receive the lab results over the next several weeks, but when none arrived I called her.

Andrea's voice was positively scathing. "No, I didn't go in for any of your ridiculous tests. I decided they weren't necessary. I went to an iridologist instead [iridology is an alternative field that makes diagnoses by examining the iris of the eye]. He looked in my eyes and told me everything was all right. I just need to have my colon cleaned out, he said. I did it, and now I feel great. All my symptoms went away. So I don't need your kind of medicine. I thought you were an alternative doctor, but you're just like all the rest of them!" With that she hung up.

Because I want so much to be all things to all people, I felt badly. I thought I had made it clear to Andrea that the tests were only for safety's sake. From the point of view of prudence, an iridologist's clean bill of health is worthless. There is no hard evidence behind iridology. The field is based mostly on intuition.

Intuition and prudence are opposites. Each has its place, but they are not interchangeable principles. People buy houses based on affinity, feel, or the principles of feng shui (traditional Chinese rules of architecture), but they check for termites by having inspectors crawl around the foundation. Prudence is a matter of the tangible, the anxious, and the careful. It is the guiding philosophy of conventional medicine, which does nothing but crawl under anatomical foundations. Iridology, like all of natural medicine, depends on feel rather than on fact. It may possibly be useful as a guide to treatment, but it is not a warranty against serious diseases.

I include this little lecture here because I could not give it to Andrea. She had hung up on me. It was in a sour mood that I turned to my next appointment.

David, a thirty-eight-year-old widower with two children, complained of a spastic colon and constipation. Over the years he had suffered from this problem occasionally, generally in association with periods of stress.

"How do you want me to approach this, David?" I asked, wishing to avoid another Andrea. "Shall I be a medical doctor or an alternative practitioner? I don't think I can be both at once."

"As an alternative doctor," he answered, without hesitation. "I want treatment, not a bunch of tests."

I said that I would try to help, but reiterated that I would not be providing the conventional medical service of looking out for any serious diseases he might have. David said he understood, and promised to use his regular physician if he felt the need to rule out anything dangerous.

Over the next couple of months, we worked on stress reduction, dietary changes, and modification of bowel habits. David's constipation rapidly improved for a while, but returned during a period of particularly high stress at work. Then, just before Christmas, David told me he had found some blood in his stool.

A warning bell went off in my head. I felt compelled to tell David that although a spastic colon can cause bleeding, cancer was another possibility. Medically speaking, he needed a sigmoidoscopic exam. I recommended a good gastroenterologist.

David asked me whether cancer was likely. I had to admit that at his young age and with his twenty-year history of strict vegetarianism, colon cancer was improbable. But I also pointed out that even a 1 percent chance feels a lot like 100 percent if it happens.

After thinking about it carefully, David said that he did not want to waste his time on a series of unpleasant and expensive tests whose likelihood of finding anything was very low. I agreed that such a decision was in his hands—as long as he understood that I had not made him any promises of safety.

David soon stopped seeing me. He decided to receive colon cleansing treatments. When he did not call back for six months, I assumed that he had found satisfaction at the colonic hygienist's office.

Then, one late spring morning, David called, sounding weak and worn. "I need your opinion, Dr. Bratman, on whether I should get chemotherapy."

I was thunderstruck. Why was he getting chemotherapy? It developed that he had been bleeding occasionally the entire time he was getting colonics, but hadn't told the colon therapist. He hadn't called the gastroenterologist until the bleeding became severe. Sigmoidoscopy revealed a colon cancer the size of an orange.

Shamefully, I must admit that my first thought was for my own safety. Had I committed malpractice? Grief followed a few seconds later. Who would take care of his two children?

I visited David in the hospital. He looked thinner than usual, almost transparent, and as he moved from bed to chair, I noticed his legs tremble. Yet, I could find no trace of depression or anxiety. David glowed with the light that is sometimes released by disaster, and said that his colon hygienist felt utterly confident that he could beat the cancer.

On questioning, his oncologist informed him that chemotherapy and radiation did not offer any reasonable hope of a cure. So David decided to take herbs and supplements instead and go on a special anticancer diet. He also practiced visualizations with enthusiasm and vigor. By the week prior to his death, David had arrived at a deep state of acceptance. His will to live changed into a will to bless, and the light of his face was beautiful. He died on Christmas morning, just over a year after he first saw blood in his stool.

I wondered whether I should have refused to treat David. I could have insisted he see a gastroenterologist. Had I so insisted, he might have complied.

However, I hate to coerce my patients. I refuse to play power games. I have built my whole practice on consultation, on equality, and on patient responsibility. But did I lull him into complacency by going along with his desire for alternative treatment? Would he have survived with a six months jump on the cancer?

Through many experiences like this one, conventional medical doctors become very compulsive. I recommend that patients appreciate this compulsiveness, and use it for what it offers, rather than criticize it for its lack of faith.

CONCLUSION:
THE BEST OF BOTH WORLDS

The preceding pages presented the relative strengths and weaknesses of alternative and conventional medicine. Armed with this information, it is possible to make health care choices that represent the best of both worlds. The general technique is simple to state: Use every form of medicine where it is strongest.

Perhaps this approach is best illustrated through a story. One that comes to mind is that of a thirty-five-year-old accountant named Susan. Unerringly, she played to the strong suit of each health care method whose aid she sought, and successfully avoided trusting recommendations that were not worthy of trust. Her method of navigating the worlds of alternative and conventional medicine presents an ideal model for those who would do the same.

Over several months Susan had developed increasing symptoms of abdominal discomfort. The chiropractor whom she had been seeing for neck pain promptly diagnosed a "stuck" ileocecal valve. But Susan wasn't sure if she could trust him.

Instinctively recognizing that conventional medicine is better at diagnosis than alternative medicine, she decided to seek the opinion of a medical doctor. A gastroenterologist named Dr. Blossom performed a series of tests, some of them quite unpleasant, and ultimately diagnosed Crohn's disease. He then recommended that she take a certain drug.

Crohn's disease is a little-understood condition that involves inflammation of various parts of the intestines. Its symptoms can vary from mild to severe, and it can have life-threatening complications. Susan's case was mild.

Susan intuitively understood that her doctor had recommended drug treatment automatically, as a matter of course. She had heard the old saying, "If what you hold is a hammer, all problems will seem like nails." Reasoning from this, she recognized that doctors naturally tend to prescribe drugs even when they are not absolutely necessary.

But Susan knew that it is better to avoid medications whenever reasonably possible. Therefore, she asked the physician to tell her whether it was absolutely essential that she take the recommended treatment. At first, Dr. Blossom insisted on it, but, on respectful questioning, he admitted that for such a mild a case drugs were not absolutely necessary. He just thought they would make her feel better.

Susan thanked the doctor for his good intentions. Then she asked how she could determine when taking the medication might become urgent. Dr. Blossom gave her a list of signs and symptoms that would indicate an absolute need for drug therapy. Susan wrote these down and promised to return if she developed any warning signs of increasing danger. She would return for twice yearly examinations anyway, to make sure she wasn't getting into trouble.

Next, Susan considered which form of alternative medicine she wanted to try. She chose acupuncture, because it seemed to her that it was the most comprehensive alternative approach to healing available. After carefully searching out a highly skilled acupuncturist, Susan made an appointment. The acupuncturist, Dr. Kim, examined her extensively from the Chinese point of view. Then, he treated her with Chinese herbs and weekly acupuncture sessions. Soon all the symptoms of Crohn's disease disappeared.

Susan kept up her regular checkups with Dr. Blossom for years. The physician grudgingly admitted that he was impressed with her progress. One particularly stressful year, however, Susan's Crohn's disease got out of hand. Mild discomfort developed into intense pain, accompanied by nausea, fever, and bloody diarrhea. Acupuncture couldn't control the symptoms. So she returned to Dr. Blossom ahead of schedule.

With a triumphant look of "I told you so," Dr. Blossom prescribed drug therapy. "If you had followed my advice," he went on to lecture, "this would never have happened to you."

Refusing to get defensive, Susan asked dispassionately, "Are you sure it wouldn't have happened? Does drug therapy have the power to prevent all flare-ups?" If the answer was yes, she thought she might decide to stay on drugs permanently. She didn't like being in this much pain.

But again the physician backed down. "Actually, now that you ask me directly, I must admit that flare-ups like these can happen anyway, even if you are taking prophylactic medication."

Susan graciously avoided making anything out of this small victory. She simply took the prescribed medication with gratitude. When the disease calmed down, she switched back to acupuncture and herbal treatment, and has remained well through the time of this writing—four more years.

Susan's story is a perfect example of the intelligent combined use of alternative and conventional medicine. She prudently used conventional medicine for diagnosis and treatment of acute symptoms. But she turned to alternative medicine for long-term maintenance, thereby minimizing the use of potentially toxic drugs.

At no point did she get angry at her practitioners, whether alternative or conventional. She was always gracious and grateful, but she didn't accept anyone's advice as the absolute truth. Susan simply listened, asked intelligent questions, and retained the ultimate responsibility for her own health care. Understanding that her chiropractor might not recognize the limits of his own ability to make diagnoses, she sought a more precise analysis from a medical doctor. Similarly, she recognized that a conventional doctor would likely prescribe drugs too freely, and questioned Dr. Blossom closely regarding their necessity.

When her condition got out of control, however, Susan understood that conventional medicine is often the best option for severe symptoms. When the crisis was over, Susan returned to the gentler options of alternative medicine. Through following such a course as Susan's, it is possible to get the best of both worlds.

SECTION V

RECOMMENDATIONS BY ILLNESS

The following section lists a number of common conditions and recommends those methods most likely to prove helpful.

Note: I deliberately do not give dosages for all the herbs and supplements I recommend below, for in some cases dosages must be individualized. In the case of standardized herbal extracts, I give the dose by the constituents to which the extracts have been standardized.

In general, it is best to consult with a qualified alternative health care practitioner. I also advise consultation with a conventional medical doctor to rule out serious underlying disease.

ANXIETY

Effectiveness of alternative methods for this condition: Moderate

The simple intervention of cutting down on sugar and caffeine can sometimes diminish overall anxiety remarkably. Among food supplements, the most generally useful is GABA. This nonessential amino acid can be quite effective when taken on a daily basis at a dose of 750–1,000 mg.

Standardized extracts of the herb kava can also reduce anxiety. The dose taken should provide 45–70 mg of kavalactones three times daily. Acupuncture is sometimes very effective for anxiety, and sometimes not. Massage can be helpful if received frequently.

ARTHRITIS (Osteoarthritis, not rheumatoid)

Effectiveness of alternative methods for this condition: Poor to excellent

Acupuncture sometimes has dramatic pain-relieving effects in cases of arthritis, and these may be prolonged. Chinese herbology may also be beneficial, especially for the type of arthritis that varies in intensity with the weather. As always, a trained Chinese herbologist is necessary for proper use of this complex art.

The Western herb devil's claw occasionally helps people with arthritis. The most famous supplement treatment for this problem is glucosamine sulfate. In my experience, glucosamine sulfate at a dose of 500 mg three times daily helps about half the arthritis sufferers who try it. Boron is sometimes packaged with glucosamine sulfate to improve effectiveness.

Some people experience dramatic relief from arthritis by identifying and avoiding allergenic foods.

ASTHMA

Effectiveness of alternative methods for this condition: Poor to moderate

The most generally useful dietary modification for asthma is to eliminate milk from the diet. This single intervention is often quite effective, especially in children, but it must be given a month to work. Cheese and yogurt don't matter so much. This is because it is the proteins in the skim part of the milk that cause allergic reactions. In cheese and yogurt, these proteins have been partly digested by bacteria.

The most frequently recommended food supplements include quercitin, magnesium, betaine HCL before meals, vitamin C, and vitamin B6. Of all these, quercitin is the most often helpful, taken at a dose of 500 mg three times daily. Still, it doesn't succeed very often.

Vitamin B12 injections are sometimes remarkably effective for mild asthma, especially in children. However, conventional asthma inhalers are less invasive and fairly safe if used correctly.

Grindelia, stinging nettles, ephedra, and lobelia are Western herbs commonly recommended for asthma, but their success rate is not impressive. Chinese herbal treatment is effective somewhat more often, but, as always, this requires a good Chinese herbologist. Acupuncture is only occasionally helpful for asthma.

BLADDER INFECTIONS

Effectiveness of alternative methods for this condition: Moderate to excellent

The most generally useful herb is uva-ursi, or bearberry. It is commonly packaged with other herbs such as juniper, cleavers, and parsley. This treatment is quite effective when used at the onset of bladder infections, or in a single prophylactic dose after intercourse. It can also be used continually for prevention. However, herbal treatment does not usually resolve an infection that has really "settled in." The dose of standardized uva-ursi taken should supply 50–100 mg of arbutin three times daily.

Cranberry juice can be helpful too, but it is important not to confuse cranberry juice cocktail with the real article. Cranberry cocktail is only a few percent cranberry juice. True cranberry juice tastes terrible and is mainly available at health food stores. The dose is 8 ounces a day. Cranberry extract is also effective, and it is easier to take in the substantial doses necessary to achieve a full effect. It is better for prevention than for the treatment of actual infections.

These herbal treatments often work for irritable bladder too—symptoms of a bladder infection without any bacteria present.

CANCER

Effectiveness of alternative methods for this condition:
Prevention—excellent; Treatment—unknown

Epidemiological studies have proven that a low-fat, semivegetarian diet dramatically decreases the incidence of all the major forms of cancer. Even some medical authorities have wondered aloud whether as a society we shouldn't be spending more effort on cancer prevention than on treatment. A general improvement of the typical U.S. diet would save an immense amount of money, not to mention suffering.

Alternative medicine also has a definite use alongside conventional cancer treatment. In particular, acupuncture is often used to reduce the side effects of chemotherapy. Herbs, massage, and dietary support can be helpful as well.

Many alternative techniques are promoted as useful in the treatment of cancer too, but this is a much more controversial issue. I am not so foolish as to recommend any of the well-known alternative cancer treatments while I still carry on a private practice. Medical boards behave aggressively toward doctors who provide unapproved cancer therapies. Those few alternative doctors who treat cancer stay in practice only with the help of great lawyers, powerful connections, and wealthy patrons. The others soon wind up in interesting new professions like selling shoes or growing potatoes.

This vigilance is not merely a result of prejudice, as some alternative medicine activists proclaim. Actually, there is at least one excellent reason for opposing alternative cancer cures: People with cancer make an easy target for the unscrupulous. They feel desperate. If there were no regulations, the health care marketplace would be flooded with bogus cancer cures overnight.

There's a fortune to be made in the field. People with sore necks are uncomfortable, but they do not feel they must mortgage the family mansion in a desperate search for a cure. Therefore medical boards feel little need to crack down on alternative neck pain treatments.

But lingering mortal illness creates a kind of hysteria. Money loses its significance in the face of death. For this reason, society does have a legitimate responsibility to protect very sick people from exploitation by charlatans.

On the other hand, there is also such a thing as freedom of choice. If patients face death from an illness for which medical science has no cure, maybe they should have the right to try any treatment they prefer. It's their life at stake, and their money.

Proponents of alternative medicine sometimes claim that medical doctors suppress alternative cancer cures for financial reasons. The logic goes like this: If the general public discovered that treatment X cured cancer, they would stop going to doctors, and doctors would lose money.

This is the "big money" argument. I don't think it's realistic. There's big money in painkillers too, but that hasn't caused widespread suppression of acupuncture for neck pain.

The members of medical boards are mostly retired physicians volunteering to perform what they believe to be their civic duty. They regard their actions as necessary to protect the public from quacks. Their intentions are good. But there are many patients who wish the government would just get out of their way and allow them to obtain the treatments they prefer.

I believe this is one of those areas where a dynamic tension must be maintained between significant but opposing values. It is necessary to find a balance between protecting people from health care fraud and allowing them freedom of choice.

CHRONIC FATIGUE SYNDROME

Effectiveness of alternative methods for this condition: Poor to moderate

The supplement ester-C combined with bioflavonoids often improves the feeling of "flu-ishness" that accompanies this syndrome. It is often combined with the herb suma to increase energy. These two methods used together seem to help a substantial percentage of chronic fatigue sufferers. They must be used for months to reach full effectiveness.

Although they are often prescribed, echinacea and ginseng seem to make most patients with this condition worse. However, general naturopathic methods such as food allergen avoidance, lifestyle changes, and "adrenal supplementation" sometimes help.

A few patients with chronic fatigue syndrome respond to acupuncture. Chinese herbology can be useful too.

Comment: Conventional medicine recognizes the existence of this syndrome, but finds it difficult to address due to the vagueness of its symptoms. The only useful conventional treatment is antidepressants. However, conventional medical diagnosis is essential to rule out the thousands of conditions that can produce similar symptoms.

COLD SORES

Effectiveness of alternative methods for this condition: Excellent

The best alternative (or conventional) treatment for cold sores is an extract of the herb *Melissa officinalis.* It is sold as a cream under the trade name Herpilyn. In my experience it is very effective.

Supplementation with L-lysine can also prevent and treat cold sores. This method is much more effective for some people than others.

COLDS, FREQUENT OR PROLONGED

Effectiveness of alternative methods for this condition: Moderate

Chinese herbology possesses a sophisticated set of techniques for working with colds. Some are used at the first sign of a cold to stop it from occurring. In my experience these are fairly effective. Other Chinese herbal combinations are designed to be used when the patient is well, for the purpose of reducing the incidence of future infections. Still other mixtures are used for colds that will not resolve in the usual seven to ten days. As always, it takes a qualified Chinese herbalist to use these methods properly.

A mixture of the Western herbs echinacea and goldenseal is popular as a treatment for colds. It appears to be marginally effective.

The most useful dietary recommendation for frequent colds is to remove milk from the diet. This simple intervention often works. If the drop in calcium seems worrisome, simply add a calcium supplement. There may also be other trigger foods that are worth avoiding depending on the individual.

Vitamin C has been shown not to prevent colds as originally claimed. It does decrease cold symptoms modestly. Zinc also appears to be slightly helpful.

Lifestyle changes include the usual recommendations: get plenty of aerobic exercise, develop regular sleep habits, and eat well. From the mouths of both Chinese and Jewish grandmothers comes another suggestion: Keep warm! Wear a scarf!

Comment: Antibiotics do not help colds, nor have they been shown to prevent the development of complications such as bronchitis or sinus infections. Their widespread use for these conditions is a form of placebo treatment. This has been proven many times, but patients still demand antibiotics, and doctors keep on prescribing them. (Once they occur, certain complications of colds may require antibiotic treatment, although not as often as generally believed.)

DEPRESSION

Effectiveness of alternative methods for this condition: Moderate

The most famous herb for depression is St. John's wort. Some studies have shown it to be as effective as antidepressants; however, those studies involved relatively few subjects. The food supplement tyrosine is often effective for depression as well.

The method of food allergen identification and avoidance sometimes improves depression, as well. None of these treatments is as dramatically effective as Prozac.

DYSMENORRHEA (Painful Menstruation)

Effectiveness of alternative methods for this condition: Moderate to excellent

Acupuncture is often effective for dysmenorrhea, and its effect can be prolonged. A double-blind study has demonstrated that acupuncture is more effective than ibuprofen for this condition. (Ibuprofen is much cheaper, however.)

Acupuncture usually must be kept up weekly through three or four menstrual cycles to produce good results. Pain relief may last for six months or more after treatment is stopped.

Chinese herbs can often treat the pain of dysmenorrhea. They are less expensive than acupuncture and can have a long-term effect. As always, however, the services of a qualified Chinese herbalist are necessary. Chinese herbal concoctions sold in health food stores are seldom useful, because Chinese herbology demands individualized prescriptions.

The Western herb known as cramp bark has a fairly strong symptomatic effect on menstrual pain, roughly similar to that of ibuprofen, but it may cause drowsiness. It is widely available, either alone or mixed with herbs of similar reputation.

Food supplements for menstrual pain include calcium, magnesium, and vitamin E. These should be taken daily throughout the cycle for best results.

FATIGUE

Effectiveness of alternative methods for this condition: Variable

Fatigue is often very hard to treat. Dietary changes include cutting down on sugar, coffee, and fat, and identifying food allergies. The most generally useful supplements include aspartic acid (as magnesium or potassium aspartate), vitamin C, and vitamin B12 injections. However, only seldom do any of these work very well.

The Western herb suma sometimes produces a sense of increased energy after a month or two of regular usage. Regular massage, possibly because of its stress-reducing effects, can be helpful as well.

Lifestyle changes are perhaps the most important. These include: engaging in regular aerobic exercise, throwing away the TV, reducing other sedentary activities, and participating in activities that bring enjoyment. Specific exercise systems like tai chi and yoga may be useful.

Sometimes small doses of thyroid supplement can improve fatigue, even if laboratory tests show normal thyroid levels. This treatment is controversial, and the disagreement extends to which form of thyroid supplement is best to use.

Comment: In my opinion, fatigue is almost always a whole-person problem. Taking a supplement for fatigue is like putting STP oil additives in the gas tank when an automobile is sluggish. Getting a tune-up would be more to the point. Similarly, using a form of treatment that enhances overall balance is usually the best way to treat fatigue. Acupuncture and Chinese medicine may be useful in this regard.

FIBROMYALGIA

Effectiveness of alternative methods for this condition: Poor to moderate

The word *fibromyalgia* probably lumps together at least two different conditions. Depending on the underlying cause, one or another alternative method may be most useful.

The first type of fibromyalgia is like a whole-body illness. Along with symptoms of generalized muscle pain and fatigue, there may also be sleep disturbances, flulike symptoms, colon pain, headaches, and other problems. For this form of fibromyalgia, supplement therapy is usually the best treatment. Useful methods include ester-C and bioflavonoids, as well as the fibromyalgia-specific supplement malic acid. The effective dose of malic acid is 600 mg, two to four times daily.

The herb St. John's wort can help with sleep disturbances. Suma sometimes reduces fatigue.

The other type of fibromyalgia resembles a particularly severe case of ordinary chronic soft-tissue pain, and often develops after a series of auto accidents or other serious injuries. Acupuncture and the various bodywork arts (especially myofascial release) are the most generally helpful.

Comment: The expectorant guaifenesin, a constituent of most cough syrups, is also used for fibromyalgia. It can be obtained by prescription in its pure form. The protocol for using it is somewhat complicated and requires a practitioner skilled in its use.

HEADACHES

Effectiveness of alternative methods for this condition: Moderate to excellent

Acupuncture is effective for many types of headaches, and the effect can be long-lasting. Chinese herbs can be particularly useful for migraines and sinus headaches.

The Western herb feverfew is often surprisingly effective for migraine headaches of moderate intensity. The tincture is best. The dose of standardized feverfew extract taken to prevent migraines should provide about 0.25–0.5 mg of parthenolide daily. To abort a migraine, higher doses may be necessary.

The most important dietary change for headaches is cutting down on caffeine and sugar.

Chiropractic frequently relieves headaches coming from the neck. For headaches that follow a blow to the head (post-traumatic headaches), cranial osteopathy is the best approach. However, it is very difficult to find qualified practitioners of this subtle art.

HIGH BLOOD PRESSURE (Hypertension)

Effectiveness of alternative methods for this condition: Moderate

Lifestyle changes include weight loss, increased aerobic exercise, and the adoption of a low-fat, vegetarian diet. The most important food supplement for blood pressure reduction is coenzyme Q10. Although rather expensive, it is fairly effective for mild to moderate hypertension and generally produces no side effects. The effective dose is 30–100 mg, three times a day. Calcium, potassium, and magnesium supplementation may be useful as well.

Standardized extracts of garlic, hawthorn, and khella can significantly lower blood pressure too, again without side effects. Garlic must be taken in a dose that provides an "allicin potential" of 4,000 micrograms daily.

HIGH CHOLESTEROL

Effectiveness of alternative methods for this condition: Variable from poor to excellent

The most useful food supplement for cholesterol reduction is inositol hexaniacinate, known as "nonflush" niacin. It is widely used in Europe. It causes a lower incidence of side effects than does plain niacin.

Garlic, available in an odor-reduced form, can improve the ratio of "good" to "bad" cholesterol. Only standardized extracts are potent enough to produce satisfactory results. The dosage necessary is the same as in the treatment of high blood pressure. Also, an extract from the Indian myrrh tree known as guggulipid can lower total cholesterol by about 10 percent.

Recommended lifestyle changes and dietary modifications are the same as for hypertension.

INSOMNIA

Effectiveness of alternative methods for this condition: Moderate

The Western herb valerian is famous as a treatment for insomnia. Its effectiveness tends to diminish with repeated use, however. The same is also true of kava.

St. John's wort, most famous as an herbal antidepressant, also often helps insomnia when taken for several weeks.

Some individuals find acupuncture highly effective for insomnia.

IRRITABLE BOWEL SYNDROME (Spastic Colon)

Effectiveness of alternative methods for this condition: Moderate to excellent

Chinese herbology can be quite effective for this condition, especially when used in conjunction with acupuncture. The effect can last long after the treatment is stopped.

Enteric coated peppermint oil (sample product: Peppermint Plus) has been shown in double-blind studies to produce symptomatic relief of irritable bowel pain.

Food allergy treatment may be helpful too, although there is always the danger of the food allergy spiral (see the discussion of food allergies in chapter 4).

MENOPAUSE AND OSTEOPOROSIS

Effectiveness of alternative methods for this condition:
Menopausal symptoms: Moderate to excellent; Osteoporosis: Insufficient data

Vitamin E in a dose of 400 IU (international units) daily has been shown to alleviate menopausal vaginal complaints as well as hot flashes. Another popular supplement is gamma-oryzanol, or ferulic acid. This extract of rice bran has been shown to alleviate many menopausal symptoms.

A high dietary intake of soybean-based foods may also be helpful. Soybeans are rich in estrogenlike substances known as phytoestrogens. This may explain why hot flashes and other menopausal symptoms occur less frequently in China. The traditional Chinese diet is rich in soy products. Other foods containing significant quantities of phytoestrogens include celery, parsley, and most nuts and seeds.

Many herbs can alleviate hot flashes. Some of the most famous are licorice, black cohosh, and wild yam. (Note: Licorice can elevate blood pressure. A chemically altered form of licorice known as DGL is free from this side effect.) A standardized extract of black cohosh sold as Remifemin has proved beneficial for many symptoms of menopause, and is widely used for that purpose in Europe.

Dong quai is a famous Chinese herb used in many women's herbal formulas. As is typical in Chinese herbology, dong quai is meant to be combined in a personalized mixture with various other herbs. It is not supposed to be used as a "one-size-fits-all" women's tonic. Unfortunately, that is how it is often marketed in this country. It is much better to visit a qualified Chinese herbalist than to take premixed concoctions of Chinese herbs.

Acupuncture treatment may be effective for hot flashes. It can also be used to treat the emotional instability that sometimes accompanies menopause.

Comment: Many women ask me about the use of extracted plant estrogens to substitute for synthetic or animal-based estrogens. Such products are available, and they will usually alleviate symptoms of menopause. However, it is unknown whether these phytoestrogens stop osteoporosis as successfully as human estrogen does. They are only estrogenlike, so they may not do the job. Conversely, it is also possible that if human estrogens increase the risk of breast cancer, plant estrogens may do so as well.

Some authors recommend the use of estriol, DHEA, or progesterone instead of estrogen. Unfortunately, insufficient data exist to know for certain whether these hormones successfully prevent osteoporosis.

PAIN (Including Back, Neck, and Shoulder Pain)

Effectiveness of alternative methods for this condition: Moderate to excellent

Pain is one of the primary indications for alternative treatment. Reasonably good studies have demonstrated the value of acupuncture and chiropractic in many types of musculoskeletal pain. The effects may be short-lived or prolonged.

In cases of pain that does not respond to these methods, other approaches may be useful. For pain in a focalized area, myofascial release and neuromuscular techniques can be very helpful. For complex pain syndromes, muscle energy work and Rolfing can often make a significant contribution. Movement therapies such as the Feldenkrais method are particularly useful for pain that can be relieved for a time but tends to return soon.

It is of great importance to choose a good chiropractor, acupuncturist, or other practitioner. Because these are crafts, there is a big difference between the best and the worst practitioner. See chapters 9 and 10 for advice on how to identify qualified practitioners.

Comment: Conventional medicine is almost useless for most cases of soft-tissue pain. Its major value is to rule out other underlying conditions.

PROSTATE ENLARGEMENT

Effectiveness of alternative methods for this condition: Excellent

A standardized extract of the saw palmetto berry is widely used in Europe for the treatment of benign prostatic hypertrophy, with excellent results. The effective dose should provide about 145 mg of fatty acids and sterols, twice a day. Zinc supplementation can also help, but excessive doses of zinc can be toxic.

RESTLESS LEGS SYNDROME

Effectiveness of alternative methods for this condition: Excellent

Acupuncture is highly effective for restless legs syndrome. In my experience, three to six sessions of acupuncture at weekly intervals usually suffice to make the restlessness diminish significantly. The treatments can then be spaced progressively further apart, and finally stopped altogether, with no loss of effect.

Besides acupuncture, a number of dietary supplements sometimes relieve this problem. These include calcium, magnesium, potassium, iron, folic acid, L-tryptophan, and vitamin E.

Caffeinated beverages tend to increase muscle tension, and thus may exacerbate this condition. Similarly, excessive consumption of sugar may produce restlessness in those susceptible to hypoglycemia.

SERIOUS CHRONIC ILLNESSES

Effectiveness of alternative methods for these conditions: Generally low

Deep internal problems such as chronic hepatitis, multiple sclerosis, and lupus are very difficult to treat by any means, including conventional medicine. The best results I have seen have been with Chinese herbs and acupuncture.

For serious illnesses, it is absolutely essential to seek out the most qualified practitioners available. A run-of-the-mill acupuncturist or herbologist will probably provide little to no help.

Food allergen identification and avoidance can sometimes cure severe illnesses.

A powerful, mysterious illness that can't be diagnosed by conventional medicine, or a standard illness that, for no obvious reason, fails to respond as expected, often indicates the presence of a deep psychological process. Body-oriented psychotherapy may help, such as process work, Hakomi, bioenergetics, or Reichian therapy. (See the section in chapter 8 called "Body-Oriented Psychotherapy.")

Sometimes mysterious illnesses respond to very simple interventions, such as removing mercury fillings from teeth or using digestive enzymes, but not often.

TENDINITIS

Effectiveness of alternative methods for this condition: Moderate

Acupuncture, especially electric acupuncture, is often highly effective for tendinitis. Neuromuscular therapy and myofascial release can also be helpful, but sometimes they worsen the problem. Resting the affected tendon is always important.

VARICOSE VEINS

Effectiveness of alternative methods for this condition: Moderate

The herbs gotu-kola and butcher's-broom can often help varicose veins. The dose of a standardized extract of gotu-kola should provide 24–48 mg of asiaticoside daily. Standardized butcher's-broom should supply 16.5–33 mg of ruscogenins three times daily

RESOURCES

BIBLIOGRAPHY

Because so many good books have been written on the various aspects of alternative medicine, it is not possible for me to review more than a small percentage. The books listed below are some of my personal favorites.

An excellent guide to the whole spectrum of available information is *Redwing Reviews,* published by the Redwing Book Company, 44 Linden St., Brookline, MA 02146. They may be reached by phone at 1-800-873-3946, or over the Internet at redwing@oa.net. While Redwing specializes in books relating to acupuncture and Oriental medicine, the company's seventy-page catalog contains thumbnail sketches of excellent books from all departments of alternative medicine.

General Naturopathic Methods

The Encyclopedia of Natural Medicine, by Michael Murray, N.D., and Joseph Pizzorno, N.D., Prima Publications, 1991. This text is a complete and comprehensive guide to naturopathic medicine written for the layperson. Its style is serious, reflective, and accurate. Although Murray and Pizzorno are among the most conscientious of naturopathic authors, they do not always carefully distinguish between solid science and loose speculation.

Back to Eden, by Jethro Kloss (multiple publications in the public domain). A classic work of traditional naturopathic thinking, Kloss's book captures in its style and content the full flavor of the original nineteenth-century movement. There is no science here—just an exuberant love of the natural life.

Food Supplements

Healing with Food: Two Hundred Eighty-One Nutritional Plans for Fifty Common Ailments, by Melvyn Werbach, M.D., Harper Collins, 1994. Werbach is the author of one of the preeminent textbooks on nutritional medicine, but this one is written for the layman. It is perhaps mistitled. While it does address food per se to some extent, it is most useful as a guide to food supplement treatment.

The Encyclopedia of Nutritional Supplements, by Michael Murray, N.D., Prima Publications, 1996. This book is a comprehensive guide to the whole range of food supplement treatments.

Herbs

Standardized Herbal Extracts:
The Healing Power of Herbs, by Michael Murray, N.D., Prima Publications, 1995. Here again, Murray presents information that is both well-researched and grounded in clinical realities. This book is a source of solid information on the proven uses and risks of numerous standardized herbal extracts.

Raw Herbs

Rodale's Illustrated Encyclopedia of Herbs, Rodale Press, 1987. This compendium of herb lore also contains up-to-date scientific information about the uses and dangers of herbal treatment. However, it is more of an encyclopedia than a practical guide. The editors seldom make actual recommendations for treatment.

Herbal Healing for Women, by Rosemary Gladstar, Fireside Books, 1993. Gladstar is a strong advocate of the traditional principles of herbology, and an opponent of those who would make herbology a branch of Western science. This book is grounded in her extensive knowledge, considerable clinical experience, and deep love for herbs. However, its philosophical point of view will not appeal to everyone.

School of Natural Healing, by John Christopher, Christopher Publications, 1996. This is one of the classic American works on herbology by an acknowledged master. It organizes herbal treatments into categories, and also includes reams of classic naturopathic advice. Like Gladstar's, this book is nearly free from science.

Dietary Therapy

Staying Healthy with Nutrition, The Complete Guide to Diet and Nutritional Medicine, by Elson Haas, M.D., Celestial Arts Press, 1991. Written by the author of the classic *Staying Healthy with the Seasons,* this book is a well-rounded and comprehensive approach to the subject of nutrition.

Healing with Whole Foods: Oriental Tradition and Western Nutrition, by Paul Pitchford, North Atlantic, 1994. In this book, Pitchford attempts to unite the Oriental and Western approaches to diet. His synthesis is impressive, if not absolutely convincing.

The Complete Guide to Food Allergy and Intolerance, by Jonathon Brosoff, M.D., and Linda Gamlin, Crown Publishing, 1992. This is a good introduction to a popular dietary method. It delves into the theory behind food allergy and sensitivity treatment as well as the practicalities of applying it. Like all books on the subject, however, it fails to warn against the most common side effect of this treatment: the frequent development of an obsession with food.

Homeopathy

The Science of Homeopathy, by George Vithoulkas, Grove Weidenfeld, 1980. This book is still one of the most well respected texts on classical or traditional homeopathy. Vithoulkas is a recognized contemporary master of the subject. His comprehensive presentation includes both philosophical and practical advice.

Homeopathic Medicine at Home, by Maesimund Panos, M.D., Jeremy Tarcher/Putnam, 1981. In contrast to Vithoulkas's book, this is a guide to what may be called symptomatic homeopathy, a nontraditional approach that is useful for self-treatment. Panos covers homeopathic treatments for many common medical conditions.

Chinese Medicine

The Web That Has no Weaver: Understanding Chinese Medicine, Ted Kaptchuk, O.M.D., Congden & Weed, 1993. This remains the best serious introductory book on acupuncture and Chinese medicine. Kaptchuk is extremely bright, and his analysis is nontrivial. The first several chapters are masterpieces of exposition, explaining the important features of Chinese medicine in a way that is both understandable and deep. Later chapters become somewhat technical and will probably strain the patience of a lay reader.

Bodywork

Massage:

Complete Book of Massage, by Hudson Clare Maxwell, Random House, 1988. Maxwell's book provides a comprehensive guide to the principles of massage, integrating all major approaches from around the world.

Zen Shiatsu, by Shizuto Masunago and Wataru Ohashi, Japan Publications, 1993. One of the best available introductions to Shiatsu, or Japanese acupressure massage, this book is profusely illustrated and clearly written.

Movement Therapy:

Awareness Through Movement, by Moishe Feldenkrais, Harper San Francisco, 1991. This is Feldenkrais's most accessible book on the method that bears his name. It contains both a summary of the philosophic underpinnings of the Feldenkrais technique as well as many useful practical exercises. While it is not a substitute for an actual Feldenkrais practitioner, it is a good introduction to this sophisticated bodywork method.

Rosen Method of Movement, by Marion Rosen and Sue Brenner, North Atlantic Books, 1991. This is a beautifully written and illustrated book that successfully explains the basic elements of Rosen movement therapy. It also contains many specific hints that can be used without further individual instruction.

The Alexander Technique, by John Gray, St. Martin's Press, 1991. The Alexander technique is a unique approach to bodywork, well introduced by Gray in this book.

Body/Mind Medicine

Mind/Body Medicine, edited by Daniel Goldman, Ph.D., Consumer Reports Books, 1993. Goldman presents a good survey of the basic methods used to treat illnesses through the mind. He adequately covers stress reduction, visualizations, and positive thinking, including both practical hints and fascinating tidbits from the developing science of psychoneuroimmunology.

Working with the Dreaming Body, by Arnold Mindell, Viking Penguin, 1989. Mindell is the founder of a sophisticated form of body-oriented psychotherapy. Although none of Mindell's books do justice to his highly experiential methods, this one is perhaps the most accessible. It introduces Mindell's concept that symptoms are dreams in the body, and gives some hints as to how this insight can be used to treat physical problems.

Healing into Life and Death, by Stephen Levine. Anchor Press/Doubleday, 1989. After Elisabeth Kübler-Ross, Stephen Levine is probably the most well known advocate of work with the dying. But his sensitive and compassionate approach does not distinguish between terminal and nonterminal illnesses; as Levine says, we are all terminal. This book offers a universal approach to healing in depth.

Body-Centered Psychotherapy: The Hakomi Method, Ron Kurtz, LifeRhythm, 1990. Hakomi is one of the most impressive of the mind/body approaches. In this useful book, Kurtz gives a clear introduction to the system of healing he pioneered.

Holistic Medicine

Health and Healing, by Andrew Weil, M.D., Houghton Mifflin, 1995. This is a fairly balanced and intellectually stimulating analysis of conventional and alternative medicine. Dr. Weil is most interested in the body's ability to heal itself.

General Naturopathy

American Association of
  Naturopathic Physicians
P.O. Box 20386
Seattle, WA 98102
(206) 323-7610

Bastyr University
144 N.E. 54th St.
Seattle, WA 98105
(206) 523-9585

Herbs

American Herbalist Guild
P.O. Box 1683
Soquel, CA 95073

The Herb Research Foundation
1007 Pearl St., #200
Boulder, CO 80302
(303) 443-0949

Sage (Rosemary Gladstar's
  Educational Foundation)
P.O.,Box 420
E. Barre, VT 05649
(802) 479-9825

Acupuncture and Oriental Medicine

The American Academy of Medical
  Acupuncture (AAMA)
5820 Wilshire Blvd., Suite 500
Los Angeles, CA 90036
(213) 937-5514

(**Note:** This organization certifies medical doctors who practice acupuncture. The number of training hours the AAMA requires of its members is much lower than what the AAAOM requires of nonphysician acupuncturists, but it is better than nothing. In most states, medical doctors can legally practice acupuncture with no training in it at all. Membership in this organization guarantees a certain minimal level of training.)

American Association of Acupuncture and
  Oriental Medicine (AAAOM)
433 Front St.
Catasauque, PA 18032
(610) 433-2448

National Commission for the
  Certification of Acupuncturists
  (NCCA)
P.O. Box 97075
Washington, DC 20090-7075
(202) 232-1404

Massage Therapy

American Massage Therapy Association
820 Davis St., Suite 100
Evanston, IL 60201
(708) 864-0123

Rolf Institute
P.O. Box 1868
Boulder, CO 80306-1868
(303) 449-5903

Chiropractic

American Chiropractic Association
1701 Clarendon Blvd.
Arlington, VA 22209
(703) 276-8800

Movement Therapy

Feldenkrais Guild
P.O. Box 489
Albany, OR 97321-0143
(541) 926-0981

Hellerwork, Inc.
406 Berry St.
Mt. Shasta, CA 96067
(916) 926-2500

The Pilates Studio
29 W. 56th St.
New York, NY 10019
(212) 875-0189

Cranial Osteopathy

Cranial Academy
8606 Allisonville Rd., #130
Indianapolis, IN 46250
(317) 594-0411

Body/Mind Medicine

The Academy for Guided Imagery
P.O. Box 2070
Mill Valley, CA 94942
(415) 389-9324

Biofeedback Certification Institute of
America
10200 W. 44th Ave., Suite 304
Wheatridge, CO 80033
(303) 420-2902

Process Work Center of Portland
2049 N.W. Hoyt Ave.
Portland, OR 97209
(503) 223-8188
(This center provides training and certification in Arnold Mindell's approach.)

Miscellaneous

American Holistic Medical Association
4101 Lake Boone Trail, #201
Raleigh, NC 26707
(919) 787-5146

INDEX

migraine headaches, 44, 110, 117, 130-131, 205-206
milk thistle, 76
milk, avoiding, 232, 236
Mindell, Arnold, 191-195
miraculous cures, 97-98
Morton's neuroma, 117
movement therapies, 161-171
multiple sclerosis (MS), 186, 244
Murray, Michael, N.D. 91
muscle energy manipulation, 142, 173, 242-243
myofascial pain syndrome, 143
myofascial release, 143, 173, 242

naming illnesses, Chinese versus conventional medicine, 112-115
National Commission for the Certification of Acupuncturists (NCCA), 115, 254
national sanitation movement, 30
natural medicine 9-11, 17. *See also* naturopathy.
natural vitamins, 85
nature cure, 60
nature doctors, 60
nature, improving on, 61
naturopathy, 8, 33, 51-52, 59-98
neck pain, 117, 145
    chiropractic treatment for, 151
    cranial osteopathy effective for, 183
negative placebo effect, 14
nerve outflows, 152
neuromuscular technique, 141-142, 242
niacin, 84
    "nonflush," 81
Nutritional Influences on Illness, 78, 83
nutritional medicine, 79

obsession, diet becoming, 93-94
organic foods, 87
Oriental medicine. *See* Chinese medicine.
orthorexia nervosa, 93-94
osteopathic medicine, 174
osteoporosis, 241

PABA, 84
pain, 242-243
    "it's all in your head", 164
    musculoskeletal, 22, 32, 36
    treatment of, 242-243
    why it persists, 164-168
Palmer, Daniel, 152
paranoia vs. trust, 221-226
Pauling, Linus, 67
peppermint, 76, 241
peripheral neuropathy, 117

phenylalanine, 84
physical examination in Chinese medicine, 123
physical therapy, 32, 139
phytoestrogens, 242
Pilates, 162
Pizzorno, Joseph, 91
placebo effect, 14, 38, 43-45
plantar fasciitis, 117, 143
positive thinking, 190-191
posture, Rolfing effects on, 145
pragmatic crafts, 105
Preissnitz, Vincent, 60
pretend science, 28
prevention of illnesses, 29-31, 35, 86, 118
Primary Respiratory Mechanism, 175
Process Oriented Psychotherapy (Process Work), 185, 191-195
prostate, 243
provings, homeopathic, 100
Prozac, 237
psoas muscle, 148
psychotherapy, body oriented. *See* body-oriented psychotherapy
Psychotherapy, Process Oriented. *See* Process Oriented Psychotherapy
pulse in acupuncture, 128

Qi, 18, 33-34
quackery, 39-41

radical diets, 19, 94
raw foods theory, 18, 88
raw herbs, 74-75
referrals, good sources of, 208-209
refined foods, 85
Reich, Wilhelm, 191
Reichian therapy, 244
reliability of treatments, 42
Remefemin, 242
research, double-blind, 38. *See also* individual alternative methods.
    funding problems in alternative medicine, 52, 74, 78, 122
responsible treatment, keeping patients from, 40-41
restless-legs syndrome, 243
Rolfe, Ida, 143-145
Rolfing, 32, 34, 143-145, 243
    costs, 34
Rolfing Movement Integration, 162
romanticism, 18
rose hips, 85
Rosen method, the, 146
rotator cuff tear, 142